"Zowie! One of my favorite herbal authors hits a home run again! I didn't know you could do so many things with herbs. Pip Waller stretches the herbal imagination!"

MATTHEW WOOD, herbalist and author of *The Book of Herbal Wisdom*

❧

"Another wonderful, very useful, and incredibly beautiful book from Pip Waller."

STEPHEN BUHNER, herbalist, earth poet, and award-winning author of *The Lost Language of Plants*

❧

"Pip, a successful and experienced herbalist, has put together a wonderful compendium of her own and her colleagues' favorite recipes."

ELIOT COWAN, founder of the Blue Deer Center, New York, and author of *Plant Spirit Medicine*

❧

"This is an amazing resource full of recipes for a wide variety of daily living and healing products. Great for our health and the environment! I recommend it to anyone who wants to live well and develop a deeper relationship with the products that they use."

MICHAEL VERTOLLI, founder of the Living School of Herbalism, Canada

"This book of recipes has many gems, which will delight everyone from experienced professional herbalists to herb-loving beginners. A truly creative and inspirational book."

LUCY HARMER, author of *Shamanic Astrology*

❧

"Having known Pip for approaching thirty years, her ongoing commitment to herbal medicine and health care is as fervent now as it was then. Drawing on her own and colleagues' knowledge, *The Herbal Handbook for Home and Health* offers a practical, encyclopedic guide on how to make, prepare, and use home remedies."

STEVE KIPPAX, former president of the National Institute of Medical Herbalists

❧

"This essential compendium will delight and excite each and every reader, whether they are an herbalist or have a more general interest in the subject. It is an indispensible guide with easy-to-follow recipes and lovely illustrations. A must-have text for anyone interested in domestic alchemy."

DEDJ LEIBBRANDT, fellow of the National Institute of Medical Herbalists

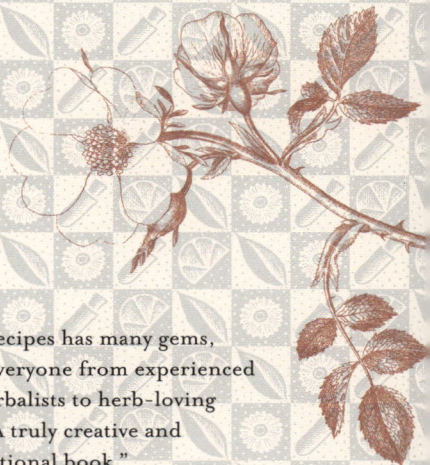

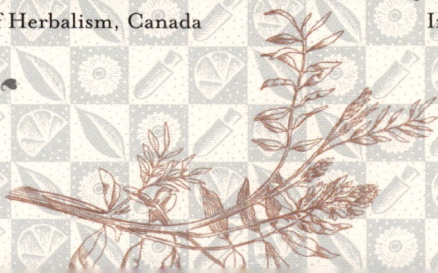

Home Herbalist

**501 RECIPES FOR
HOME, HEALTH AND HAPPINESS**

PIP WALLER

chartwell
books

Quarto

© 2024 Quarto Publishing Group USA Inc.

This edition published in 2025 by Chartwell Books,
an imprint of The Quarto Group
142 West 36th Street, 4th Floor
New York, NY 10018 USA
T (212) 779-4972 F (212) 779-6058
www.Quarto.com

Published by North Atlantic Books
P.O. Box 12327 Berkeley, California 94712
This book was conceived, designed, and produced by
Leaping Hare Press

Publisher: Susan Kelly
Commissioning: Editor Monica Perdoni
Senior Editor: Jayne Ansell
Creative Director: Peter Bridgewater
Art Director: Wayne Blades
Cover Designer: Angelika Piwowarczyk
Interior Designer: Andrew Milne

Color Origination by Ivy Press Reprographics

ISBN: 978-0-7858-4908-7

Printed in China

CONTENTS

Chapter One

The Power of Plants

HERBAL LORE BELONGS TO US ALL, A GREAT AND LASTING LEGACY. Throughout history and across cultures, plants have been used for food, shelter, clothes, and medicine. Plants contain the proteins and other nutrients that all animals need to thrive, so we depend on them for our survival. The soil itself is nourished by living plants, and even when they die, they decompose to form soil from which new plants can grow. Plants sustain all life; everything we need can be obtained from plants.

Today, however, the central role plants play in human lives has been almost forgotten in the Western world. After several generations of urbanized living, those in modern industrialized countries are far removed from nature, creating a damaging imbalance and further misuse of our greatest resource. Even most of us living in rural areas no longer regularly cultivate, gather, and use the helpful plants that grow all around us.

ALCHEMISTS OF THE NATURAL WORLD

Herbs are the wondrous "alchemists" of the natural world. They take carbon dioxide from the atmosphere for their energy production, and give back the oxygen that we need to breathe; they take nitrogen from the air and use it to make amino acids, the building blocks of proteins. Plants build all kinds of chemicals, and they do so in constant relationship to the circumstances in which they find themselves, and in communication with each other. They make medicines—for themselves, for other plants, for the soil and environment around them, and for us.

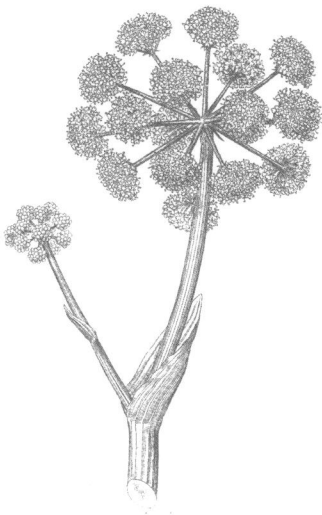

NATURAL MEDICINE

Herbal medicine has been the mainstay and root of medicine from earliest times. In some ancient tombs, archaeologists have discovered the remains of plants still known to herbalists for their power to treat conditions, such as arthritis, which modern science has detected in the bodies they accompany. Every culture and every land has a rich history of herbal medicine. Even up to the present day, many drugs used in modern medicine come from plant-based sources.

My own interest in herbal medicine grew in the 1980s, when both my parents experienced health problems. At the time, using anything other than conventional medicine was almost unheard of, and any mention of alternative medicine was met with a doubtful, "Does it actually work?" My parents were concerned, however, about the implications of medicines our regular doctor was suggesting and decided to approach an herbalist for advice. They began taking herbal remedies routinely and the results were incredible—my father was even able to avoid surgery. I was impressed and so drawn to the subject that I went on to study herbal medicine at the School of Phytotherapy in Kent, UK, and joined The National Institute of Medical Herbalists.

A NEW PERSPECTIVE

I began to learn about herbalism's rich heritage and its success in curing all kinds of problems. During the great cholera epidemic of the nineteenth century, for example, many herbalists in industrial towns became famous for rarely losing a patient; and following the disastrous explosion at Chernobyl, the Soviet nuclear plant, in 1986, it was found that growing comfrey lowered levels of radiation poisoning in the surrounding soil. This knowledge fascinated me and I continue to be enlightened.

The more I experience and learn about the power of plants, the more baffled I am that herbalism is sometimes still regarded as being paradoxically "ineffective" on the one hand and "dangerous" on the other. I wanted to write a book that would help dispel these myths and encourage readers to start their own lifelong journey of discovery into herbalism.

HARMONY & HAPPINESS

"Wood warms you three times—first when you gather it, second when you chop it, and third when you burn it."
Similarly, making your own plant-based recipes for home and health provides three sources of happiness and relaxation:

First, being outside in nature gathering plants or tending pot herbs on your windowsill, drying and preparing those you have grown, even enjoying measuring out dried herbs and oils bought in for potion making; all connect us to nature which brings harmony and balance into our lives. In fact, feeling your inherent connection to the natural world will bring inestimable happiness.

Second, pottering around in your kitchen laboratory is great fun. You will embark on an empowering journey of exploration as you discover herbs and concoct unique recipes for your home, health, and happiness.

Third, when you use the magical elixir you have made, or share it with a friend, you will feel a tremendous sense of satisfaction.

In short, plants contribute to our happiness and well-being in so many different ways; their inherent usefulness isn't the only joy they bring.

CONNECTING WITH THE NATURAL WORLD

This is a book for anyone with an interest in using plants in the home: for herbalists and kitchen herbalists, for conservationists, for anyone with even a passing interest in herbs. It's a book for those looking to live a more natural life, to welcome the spirit and usefulness of the plant world into their lives, and to connect with the natural world—whether you live in a semi-rural location (as I do) or a city apartment.

The 501 recipes in this book have been gathered by myself over years as an herbalist, and include contributions from experts across the United States, Canada, the UK, and elsewhere in Europe. They range from teas to meads, from toothpastes to face masks, from laundry detergent to air freshener. Some are simple, requiring almost no equipment; others are complex, such as cream blending, soap making, or distilling aromatic waters. My hope is that as your confidence grows, you will begin to experiment and create your own variations. The next few pages of this book are dedicated to showing you all that you need to start your plant-based preparations at home. They include equipment that you will need, information on sourcing and storing herbs, and some key techniques for preserving herbs.

Plants are truly life-enhancing, thus herbalism, and the love and appreciation of nature that it fosters, is for everyone. I hope this book helps to lead you on a rich journey of discovery.

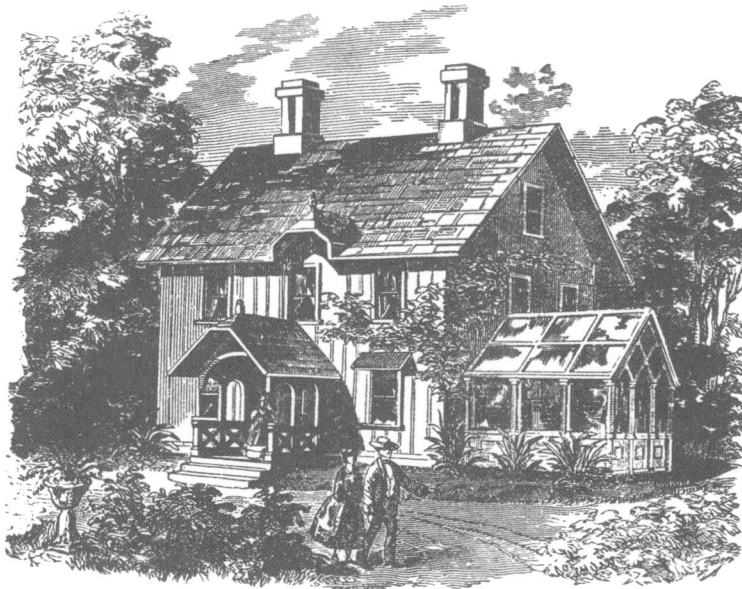

Chapter Two

Sourcing Herbs

SOURCING HERBS NEEDS A LITTLE THOUGHT. Whether you choose to pick herbs in the wild, grow your own, or buy them, you will need a certain amount of background knowledge. The following pages are dedicated to providing a few guidelines, and the Herb Directory on pages 222–243 can also be used as a starting point to help identify and source plants.

Even if you begin by buying all your ingredients, I hope that as your confidence grows you will be inspired to take a step further and discover living plants in nature. Native wisdom from all over the world states that local herbs are many times more effective than those grown at a distance. It is known that plants adapt their chemistry to their environment.

The feeling of connection that a human can have with the plant world is irreplaceable in its health-giving and balancing propensity. When you get to know living plants, you will begin to see friends everywhere you go.

PICKING HERBS IN THE WILD

Foraging, or wildcrafting, is increasingly popular, and you need not live in the woods to do it. It's amazing how many useful herbs grow in the nooks and crannies of a city. When gathering from the wild, there are a few important considerations.

First, treat the environment with respect and don't overforage. A good guideline is to always take a little under half of what is there—and if the plant is endangered, don't take any at all. If you are gathering the root of a plant, or a whole plant (as opposed to just some flowers, leaves, stems, or bark), then plant some seeds or a new plant. With some plants, you can divide the roots and replant half again.

Second, check for contamination. In farming areas, avoid land that has been crop sprayed, especially recently. In cities, find out the previous use of waste land, making sure it wasn't used for toxic chemical production, dumping, or such like. It's also important to be careful that you are not trespassing on private land, and to check local laws about gathering plants.

Plant identification is an invaluable skill, and there are excellent books with clear photographs to help the lone learner. If you take this route, you must be extremely careful not to use the wrong plant: if you're not sure, leave it alone. While few plants are seriously poisonous, some can harm and even kill you if taken by mistake. There are useful resources online about foraging; I have included some at the back of this book.

Before I pick, I follow the native tradition of asking the plant's permission in my heart (respecting a "no" if I feel I hear one), and offering gratitude and something in return. In North America, the traditional offering is tobacco; in Europe, it is oats or barley. Even if this seems strange to you, I encourage you to try it. You may be surprised at the warmth it will bring you. The earth is a living treasury, and the more you recognize its offerings, the richer your life will be.

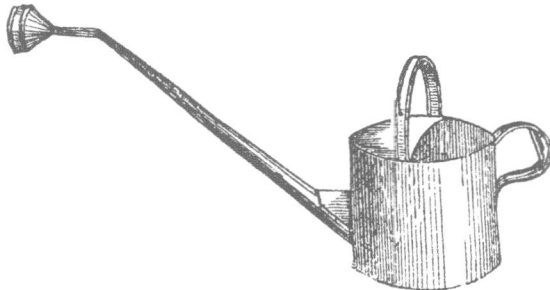

GROWING HERBS

Plants, generally, are easy to please—they like enough (but not too much) light, water, and food, and the right kind of soil. They also respond to love; talking to your plants and caring for them actually makes them grow more abundantly. This attitude can be even more important than the quality of the earth in which they are grown, as shown by the famous eco-community of Findhorn, near Forres in Scotland, who have grown impossibly enormous vegetables on soil that was little more than dirt-covered rock.

You can grow some herbs anywhere. They are ideal for urban settings and don't require a lot of space; many thrive in a windowbox or containers as well as planted in the ground. A lot of herbs—"herbs" being the general word for describing plants used in medicine, or to give flavor and texture in cooking—are especially easy to grow.

Many plants love some attention. The more you pick the flowers of the marigold, for example, the more it will flower. And most plants prefer a sheltered spot and the company of other plants. Check for any individual requirements of the herbs you grow, and grow them simply, using organic or bio methods, for maximum benefit.

Start growing whatever you feel like, and whatever you can easily find. You can sow seeds —try marigold (Calendula officinalis), nasturtium, and Californian poppy as a few easy starters.

Or buy small plants to start you off, such as oregano or marjoram, or thyme. I grow a stevia plant (a great natural sweetener) on my bathroom windowsill, where it keeps coming year after year; I keep cutting the stems to use in recipes, and more grow back. Every couple of years I repot it carefully to give it some fresh soil. I tried to grow this plant in the kitchen for a while, but the steaminess in the bathroom seems to suit her more.

Make inquiries locally to see what grows well in your area, and just try growing it. Make friends with local gardeners—they will give you tips, and probably some plants to start you off. Try planting things inside or out: if they are happy, continue as you are; if not, try something else. You will probably be pleasantly occupied and satisfied with your homegrown results.

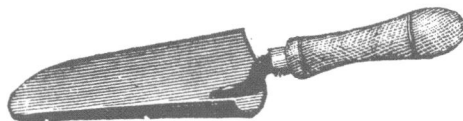

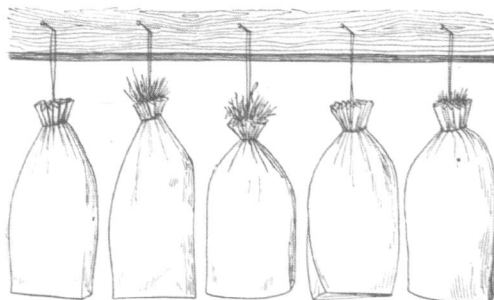

PICKING HERBS

Harvest plants on a sunny day, picking leaves and flowers around midmorning when the dew has dried. Remember to take a small pocketknife. Keep an eye on the plants you want so that you can pick them at their peak. Choose the healthiest plants or parts of plants. If you plan to use them fresh in a recipe, try to pick and use immediately.

DRYING & STORING HERBS

Wash plants, if necessary, then remove and compost unhealthy or unnecessary parts. Gather the aerial parts (those above ground) into a bundle and tie up at the bottom of the stems, or put them into a paper bag. Hang the bundle or bag in a warm, well-ventilated place, indoors or out. Herbs take up to several days to dry depending on conditions.

All parts of plants can be spread out in single layers on trays to dry in a warm, well-ventilated place. Use mesh trays or trays lined with clean dish towels or paper. Turn the plant matter daily to encourage even drying. Roots can be left whole or coarsely chopped (it's easier to cut them fresh). Flowers and leaves are easier to remove from stems when dry. You can also dry plant material in a dehumidifier.

Aim to dry the plant material enough to stop it turning moldy, without taking all the life away. Store your dried plants in paper bags sealed from the air, or in airtight jars, and keep away from direct sunlight. If dried well, herbs will keep with full properties for at least a year. After this, they will not be as beneficial.

Buying

What cannot be grown or foraged can be bought, choosing organically grown ingredients as much as possible. Be responsible when buying wildcrafted herbs, and make sure they were properly picked with sustainability in mind. Reputable suppliers of herbs can be found easily online, and you may be lucky and have a good herbal shop near enough to visit. Find a local herbal practitioner and ask his or her advice about local suppliers. This also puts you in touch with a qualified professional to consult when you need to.

When you are buying herbs in a relatively raw state—for example, dried to use in a recipe—you will easily be able to tell the quality by looking, smelling, and tasting a little.

Some of the recipes in this book include ingredients you will need to buy. All of these are readily available.

Chapter Three

Kitchen Set-Up

LITTLE SPECIAL EQUIPMENT IS NEEDED to start creating useful, plant-based preparations at home, but you will want to prepare your working area and acquire a few necessary items before you start to gather your herbs. The basic kit on pages 16–17 lists essential pieces of equipment and explains how they are used. The recipes in this book assume you have the basic kit, noting only additional "speciality" items not on this list.

Before you move on to the recipe section, you will need some knowledge of the key techniques herbalists use to extract and preserve an herb's wonderful properties. The following pages are dedicated to this, and you will be referred back to this section frequently during the course of the book.

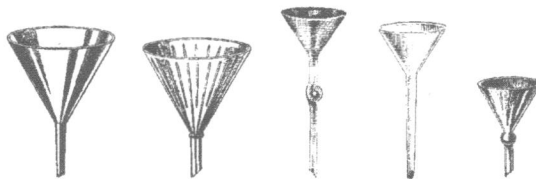

◇◇

KEY PRESERVATION TECHNIQUES

A domestic alchemist can extract and preserve the properties he or she needs from plants in various ways. The materials you choose will affect the quality of the final product. Try to choose organically grown ingredients wherever possible, and use raw (unpasteurized) honey and apple cider vinegar for anything taken inside the body. Water used for making any preparation should be of good quality; unless you have access to pure spring water, filtered is best, being both cleaner than average tap water and more environmentally friendly than bottled water.

HERBAL INFUSIONS

Leaves and flowers as well as ground roots and barks can be made into infusions (also called teas or tisanes). These can be prepared with fresh or dried herbs.

Hot Infusions

Unless instructed otherwise, teas in this book are to be made as follows:

Put 1 tsp. dried herb material or 2 tsp. fresh into a teapot or saucepan with a lid. Cover with a mug of boiling water and let sit with a lid on to infuse or brew for 10 minutes. Strain before use.

If a stronger tea is required, the traditional dose is 1 oz. dried herb or double the quantity of fresh steeped in 2⅓ cups water. Some recipes call for these stronger herbal infusions.

Cold Infusions

Cold infusions are made by steeping herbs in cold water for 2–3 hours. They are usually made with fresh flowers and leaves.

Decoctions

Parts of the plant that are tougher (such as roots and barks) need to be boiled in water. This is known as a "decoction," although it can also be called a tea. Decoctions can be made with similar amounts as the teas above, but a little extra water is added to allow for evaporation while simmering. In making decoctions, the plant matter is put into a saucepan with water, covered with a lid, heated, and then simmered for 10–15 minutes.

After the infusion or decoction is made, usually (but not always) the liquid is strained off and the solid plant matter discarded (for composting). If the liquid is being used in an eye bath or a cream, it should be strained through a strainer lined with cheesecloth or thin cotton cloth (p.16) to make sure absolutely no small parts remain.

Infusions and decoctions can be drunk hot or cold, applied externally as lotions or washes, and used in the making of other preparations, such as creams. They keep for 3 days in the refrigerator. If you bottle them hot into sterilized bottles (p.17), you can keep the unopened bottles for up to a month.

Aromatic Waters

It is exciting to turn a tea or decoction from an aromatic herb into a "water," which involves distillation. A simple method using an adapted pressure cooker is described with the recipes. Aromatic waters can keep for anywhere between 3 months and 2 years.

BASIC KIT

RACK, STRING, PAPER BAGS, SELECTION OF GLASS JARS, AND STORAGE CONTAINERS, LABELS

Freshly picked herbs can be tied together and hung from a rack to dry. When dried, store in paper bags or glass jars with tightly fitting lids, away from direct sunlight.

Jars are also used to store tinctures, vinegars, and infused oils; you may want large ones for this purpose—old candy jars work well. Small jars are useful for storing creams; bottles for liquid preparations. You may also need old shampoo bottles and so forth, plus spray bottles and dropper bottles. Almost everything you make will need a label.

Whatever you use to store your preparations needs to be particularly clean. It is absolutely essential to sterilize bottles or jars used for storing syrups, glycerin, tinctures, jellies, creams, and ointments (see box, opposite).

COFFEE GRINDER

For grinding dried herbs and roots. Ground herbs are used in infusions, oil blends, chocolates, snuff, scouring powder, medicines, and foods.

TEAPOT OR COVERED SAUCEPAN (OR A TEA INFUSER IF FOR ONE PERSON)

For brewing infusions (herbal teas).

FUNNELS

For pouring and straining. You need both large and small to fit the necks of storage bottles.

CHEESECLOTH OR THIN COTTON CLOTH

For straining potions. Use squares of cheesechloth, large cotton handkerchiefs, or dish towels.

SIFTERS AND STRAINERS

Metal sifters and strainers, from tea strainer size upward, are useful for straining. (A small wine press, of the kind normally used for home brewing, is good for pressing out tinctures, infused oils, etc.)

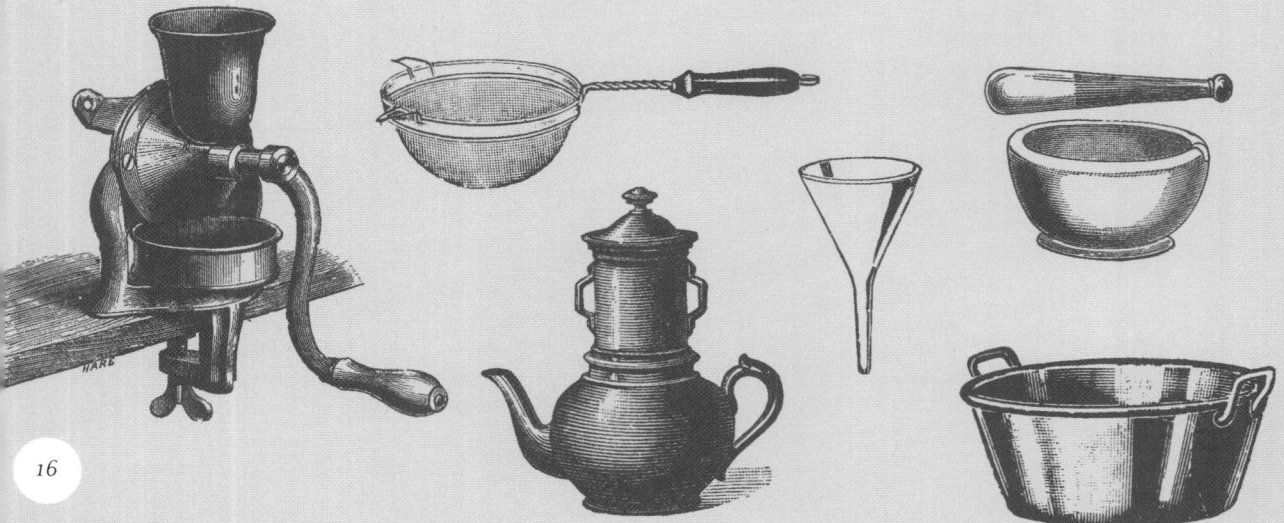

COOKING IMPLEMENTS

For brewing up mixtures, use pots, saucepans, heat-resistant stainless steel or silicone spatulas and spoons, and a potato masher.

DOUBLE BOILER/WATER BATH

For heating potions gently, use a stainless steel double boiler or a "water bath," a baking dish or saucepan filled halfway with water on the stove, with heat-resistant bowls containing your potions inside it.

MEASURING EQUIPMENT

A couple of accurate measuring cups and spoons for measuring dry and liquid ingredients. For medicinal tincture mixtures, use a narrow measuring cylinder.

DIGITAL SCALES

Some recipes require accurately weighed ingredients. Digital scales for home use can now be found in some larger department stores and online for people following weight-loss diets.

Sterilizing

It is very important to sterilize equipment properly before preserving any plant material, as failure to do so will not only lessen the shelf-life of your product, but could also potentially cause food poisoning.

Sterilize items immediately before use. Cool jars/bottles first for cold preparations, but always pour hot preparations (jellies, hot oils, syrups, etc.) into hot jars or bottles. You can sterilize items in a number of ways:

1 Remove any plastic lids and cook clean glass bottles and jars in the oven, preheated to 275°F, for 20–30 minutes.

2 Boil in water for 10 minutes (boil lids separately). Keep bottles and lids covered by water until just before use.

3 Use a microwave or dishwasher; check the manufacturer's instructions before proceeding.

The United States Department of Agriculture details safe canning methods on their website (www.usda.gov).

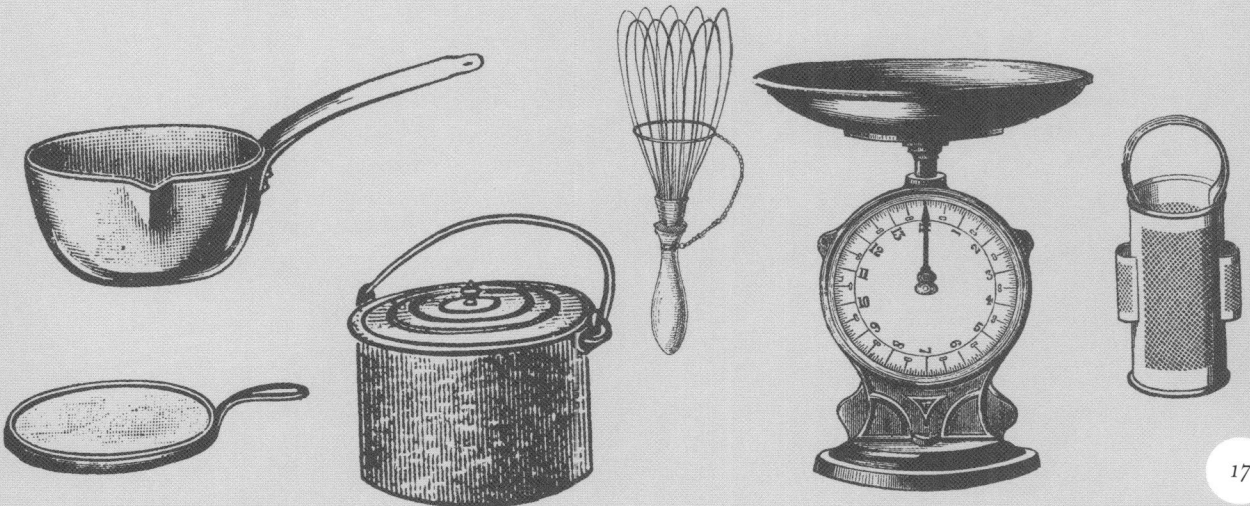

HERBAL TINCTURES

Plants' qualities can be extracted and preserved using alcohol. Tinctures, as they are known, were traditionally made by boiling herbs in wine, but are now produced by steeping the herb in a solution of alcohol and water. Herbalists use variable concentrations of alcohol for different plants, from solutions of 15–25 up to 190 proof alcohol for resins. (Resins are substances exuded from certain trees, many of which have strong antiseptic and healing properties, such as myrrh.)

Producing tinctures at home usually means using store-bought alcohol. Always aim to use organic alcohol. The best one is vodka because it has little taste, although any strong alcohol will do. Vodka is usually about 80 proof.

If you are making a tincture with fresh plant material (called a "specific tincture"), the water in the plant will even things out nicely down to a tincture of 50–60 proof. If you are using dried herbs, however, you may want to add ⅓ cup/85ml water to dilute each just over ¾ cup/200ml alcohol. Alternatively, dilute with an infusion or decoction of the herb, which gives you a combination of tea and tincture in one remedy.

Make tinctures by covering plant material with between two and five times the amount of alcohol solution in a large jar with a well-fitting lid. It is best to use weights for the amount of herb used. A general guide could be 7 oz. dried herb (10½ oz. fresh) to each 1 quart alcohol solution.

Let sit in a cool, dark place for at least 3 weeks, turning upside down or shaking the jar once a day. (Many traditions encourage talking or singing to the plants as you do this.) After 3–8 weeks, strain the liquid through a strainer or funnel lined with thin cloth. Pull the edges of the cloth up and around the macerated herbs, then twist, wring, and press it to extract all of the liquid. Store in a clean bottle.

Fluid extracts are tinctures made with equal amounts of plant material to alcohol. They can be made by double infusing (p.20).

Tinctures are used in creams, lotions, and liniments, or taken internally. Even a small dose of tincture is effective.

Some herbalists work entirely with drop doses, and some herbs are taken only in drop doses (such as 5–20 drops, 1–3 times daily); always use drop doses for children. Many herbalists use a standard adult dose of 1 tsp/5ml mixed in 2 tbsp./30ml hot or cold water, taken once a day for a tonic or preventive or 3 times a day for chronic ailments. For acute conditions, 1–2 tsp/5–10ml can be taken 3–6 times daily.

Tinctures are often mixed together in blends; there are many recipes for blends in this book. You can either buy in the tinctures to make them or produce your own, using the guidelines above. For these blends, herbalists tend to use only milliliters (ml) as measurements, as this is the easiest and best way. You can make them with teaspoon measures (1 tsp. = 5 ml, 1 tbsp. = 15ml) but it is quite fiddly. If you are regularly making these mixtures, I suggest you buy a 100ml plastic measuring cylinder (they cost about $2.50).

Not everyone can tolerate, or want to take, alcohol, in which case tinctures can be made with the same quantities of glycerin.

Many leading herbalists tailor-make tinctures each time instead of using standard amounts; as the American herbalist Matthew Wood, author of *The Book of Herbal Wisdom* (1997), explains: "I look for the distinctive taste of every plant in the extract. Therefore, I make the tincture to the 'right taste' … I prefer to think of tinctures and other preparations by analogy to wine, not to pharmaceutical drugs."

Tinctures can also be made into delicious alcoholic beverages that are pleasant to drink and have health-giving properties in small doses. These can be made with wine, mead (my personal favorite), or with any alcohol: gin (sloe gin is the famous one), brandy, vodka, rum, whiskey, if you like it, or the local home-distilled schnapps. Usually, a little honey or sugar is added while the tincture is steeping, otherwise the method is the same.

Kept in a cool place away from the sun, a well-made tincture will keep for at least 2 years, some many more.

HERBAL VINEGARS

Vinegars are a useful medium for extracting and preserving herbs; they are used in foods, taken as supplements or medicines, and used in many home-cleaning products and hair and skin tonics.

Vinegar, especially raw (unpasteurized) organic apple cider vinegar, is good for you inside and out. Taken internally, it can encourage a healthy pH balance, reduce inflammation, boost immunity, and regularize metabolism. Taken with food, it enables you to absorb minerals better. Externally, it can bring bruises to the surface, cool and reduce swellings, and benefit the hair and skin.

Herbal vinegars are made like tinctures. Steep the herb in 2–3 times the amount of vinegar. Let sit for 2–4 weeks in a cool, dark place, then strain through cloth. As medicines, the dose is the same as for tinctures (see opposite). Vinegars can keep for at least 2 years.

COMPRESS & POULTICE

Vinegars, tinctures, and teas can be used to make a compress. Soak a cloth in the herb liquid, lay it, heated or cold, against the skin, and secure with a suitable bandage. It will help to soothe aches and pains, sore throats, headaches, and skin conditions.

Fresh plant material can be used to make poultices—mashed or crushed herbs applied to the body alone. Poultices can stay in place for 2–3 days, although many choose to replace them daily.

OXYMELS

An oxymel is a tasty remedy that combines the healing properties of an herbal vinegar with honey—itself a miraculous substance, known to be antibiotic and encouraging to the immune system. Oxymels are made by gently warming an herbal vinegar with an equal amount of honey until the honey is dissolved. In sterile bottles (p.17), oxymels keep for 2 years.

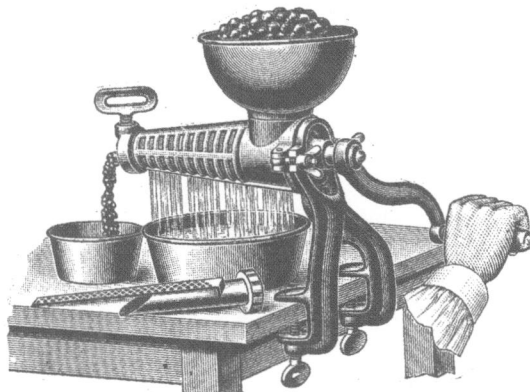

INFUSED OILS

Infused oils, made in the same way as tinctures and vinegars, can be used alone or in ointments, creams, liniments, and lotions.

To make, combine 1 part herb with 2–3 parts vegetable oil, then let sit for 4–8 weeks to infuse. Infused oils are mostly made in the shade, because vegetable oils may spoil, but some need sunlight to work properly. The recipes in this book will say if sun is required. Once infused, strain and press through cloth, as described for tinctures (p.18).

You can make an infused oil more quickly by gently heating the herb in the oil, usually in a double boiler or water bath (p.17), for 2–4 hours.

Many vegetable oils can be used to make an herbal infused oil. The most commonly used include olive, almond, sunflower, coconut, safflower, canola, grapeseed, sesame, and jojoba. The base oils all have medicinal properties of their own, and I recommend researching which oil will best offer what you require. Always use the best organically grown, cold-pressed oil that you can afford. Olive oil infusions can keep for up to a year before they start to become rancid, and coconut infusions can keep for 2 years, but most others will spoil in a few months.

Sometimes a "double infusion" is made to obtain a higher-strength product. In such cases, the infused oil is made and then used to infuse a fresh quantity of plant material. (This can also be done with tinctures, vinegars, and all water-based preparations.)

An infused oil can be made into a salve, balm, or ointment by addition of an emulsifier, such as beeswax. The more wax you use, the harder the ointment becomes. For a soft salve, 8–10 percent wax to oil is used.

LINIMENTS

Liniments are warming, stimulating rubs for aches and pains. They rub in easily and are lighter than an oil, so are useful for covering large areas. Liniments are made by mixing an infused oil and a tincture or vinegar. The two will naturally separate in the bottle, so they need to be shaken before each use. How long a liniment keeps for will depend upon the base oil (such as olive oil, almond oil) you're using.

CREAMS

Creams can be difficult to make successfully. They mix oil and water components, which require an emulsifier. The purist natural cream maker will use beeswax and a serious amount of whisking instead of a manufactured emulsifier.

To make creams the old-fashioned way, heat the oil and water components separately to a similar temperature using a double boiler or water bath (p.17); in a double boiler, you can heat the water part in the bottom and the oil in the top. Then pour the water part slowly into the oil part, whisking furiously. Once the oil and water are mixed, the cream is usually quickly cooled by placing the mixing bowl into a cold bath (a pan of cold water). Usually, you continue to whisk while cooling, and until the cream is formed, then put into sterilized jars.

Using a store-bought emulsifying wax makes cream making a simpler process. This is a substance used in cosmetic manufacturing; you can buy it made from pure vegetable sources, but because it is a "man-made" ingredient, purists tend to spurn it.

How long creams keep for varies greatly. Those made with long-lasting coconut oil, for example, could keep for a year; with some other oils, creams may last for only 1–2 months, unless a preservative is added.

SOAPS

Soap basically consists of vegetable oils that have been saponified (turned into soap) with a strong alkaloid known as lye. Soap making is easy to pull off successfully; however, it involves a lot of steps and some substances that need handling and measuring carefully. For this reason, ingredients for soaps are weighed, and you'll need a digital scale to make them.

Solid soap is made via a "cold process" using sodium hydroxide, which involves a lot of stirring and no heat. Liquid soap uses potassium hydroxide in a "hot process," which involves a lot of stirring and the use of a slow cooker to provide heat. Herbs and essential oils are then added after the oils and lye have been mixed. Soaps keep for years, but they will lose their smell over time as the essential oils evaporate.

SYRUPS, HONEYS & CANDIES

Sugar and honey can be used in various ways to preserve plants. Both can be used to make syrups that are soothing and nourishing, particularly for the throat and chest, and are good for preserving vitamin C.

A simple syrup is made by boiling a 65 percent sugar and water solution (that is, one that contains twice the quantity of sugar to liquid) for 3–5 minutes, or by first making a strong infusion or decoction and then boiling this with the sugar.

When making a syrup with raw honey, do not boil, because this destroys its healthful enzymes. Just add an equal amount of honey to a strong herbal decoction or infusion and then heat the mixture gently to dissolve. Infused honeys can also be made simply by mixing the honey and the herbs and letting infuse for a few weeks.

Store the syrup in sterilized bottles (p.17), first putting the lids on loosely, then tightening when cold. 65 percent sugar syrups keep well. You can also make a 40–50 percent syrup that will keep fairly well unopened if it is thoroughly sterilized. Syrups tend to spoil quickly once opened, so store your syrup in several smaller bottles instead of one large bottle to help improve its shelf life.

Syrups can also be sterilized again once bottled to preserve them further. Set the lids on loosely, then place the bottles on layers of paper in a saucepan (the water should reach three-quarters of the way up the bottles' sides). Simmer for 10 minutes, then immediately remove from the heat and tighten up the lids.

Candies are made from a 65 percent syrup that has been boiled for a long time. Sometimes tinctures and essential oils may be added in at the end. Some recipes use half sugar, half golden syrup or light corn syrup.

Boil the syrup for 20–30 minutes to evaporate the water, leaving more and more sugar in the mix. This then goes through several stages. The "hard-ball" stage, which is the minimum needed for candies, occurs after this 20–30 minutes, so start testing after 15 minutes. To test, drop a little of the mixture into cold water and watch.

At "hard-ball" stage, the mixture makes a ball shape; it keeps its shape but feels sticky to the touch. The next stage, known as the "soft-crack" stage, can occur minutes later. The mixture now solidifies into threads that are

21

flexible to the touch and will bend a little before breaking. The third stage, known as the "hard-crack" stage, occurs minutes after this. At this point, the threads break immediately. Because the three stages occur in quick succession, I recommend testing your mixture every few minutes after you reach the "hard-ball" stage.

Anywhere between "hard-ball" and "hard-crack" stage works for herbal candies; after that you are in burning territory. As the "hard-ball" stage is sufficient, pour your mix onto a lightly oiled baking tray when you reach this point, scoring both ways to make small lozenge shapes as it cools. Alternatively, pour into small molds and let set. If adding essential oils, do this just before pouring out. If adding honey to the mixture, I like to boil it a little longer until "hard-crack" stage is reached. Then add the honey just before pouring it out. When the contents are cold, they can be turned out and broken into pieces as necessary.

Keep the candies in a sealed container in a cool place with some confectioners' sugar, cornstarch, or ground slippery elm to stop them from sticking together. Stored this way, they will last well for 3–4 weeks and up to 6 weeks.

Essential Oils

Essential oils are a valuable addition to many recipes. These are generally bought, because they are extracted by a complex distillation process; they contain potent properties from the plant, and are used in small quantities. They mix easily in fixed oils, but tend to float on top if mixed in a water preparation, unless emulsified in some way. First mixing the oils with a little vegetable glycerin can help. Essential oils are volatile and are lost by heating, so are added at the end of any recipes using heat. Some will strip paint or eat into rubber, so if you are experimenting with recipes, keep this in mind and be cautious.

LABELING & STORING

When you have finished making a product, be sure to label it with what it is and the date made; otherwise you will end up with a shelf full of lovely potions and lotions that you have no idea what to do with.

Unless the recipe says otherwise, store all products in a cool, dark place in an appropriate vessel—a sterilized bottle or jar with a tight-fitting lid, or an airtight container. This will ensure each product keeps at its best for as long as possible. Each recipe includes a recommended shelf life; this should be used as a guide, with common sense always prevailing. If a product starts smelling odd, discard it.

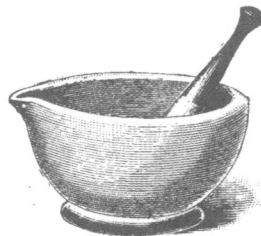

HOW TO USE THIS BOOK SUCCESSFULLY

There is a wide range of recipes in this book—from tincture blends and infusions to soaps and creams. To make them successfully, there is some important information you need to keep in mind.

INGREDIENTS

- Some recipes are made from fresh herbs, others are bought, and some use a mixture. Unless fresh or dried herbs are specified, it should be assumed that you can use *either* fresh or dried herbs for each recipe. If the amounts differ depending on whether you use fresh or dried, this will be stated.

- Many ingredients lists contain premade preparations: tinctures, infusions, and so on. Where a specific recipe for these appears in the book, you will be referred to it; otherwise, you will be referred back to the key preservations section (pp.15–22) for the standard technique.

EQUIPMENT & METHOD

- Before you start making anything, gather together the basic equipment (pp.16–17). All the recipes assume you have this equipment on hand; only if you need something less common, will it be specified.

- Some recipes are simple and others complex. In the interests of space, the various methods are described in full only once, and you will be referred back to it as required. Always carefully read the recipe and, if necessary, the general information found elsewhere in the book, before beginning.

MEASUREMENTS

- Herbalism isn't an exact science. Many herbalists do not work with rote amounts, tending to measure by eye to produce the desired result. With this in mind, most recipes—such as food, cleaners, and so on—use rough approximations.

- Some recipes, however, require that ingredients be very carefully weighed; this includes many medicines, all soaps (because you're using caustic substances), and some creams (which can be hard to make). In such recipes, cup conversions or tablespoon measurements do not provide the necessary accuracy, so they have not been provided and their use is not advised.

- Tablespoon and teaspoon measurements provided in this book are based on the following:
  1 tbsp. = 15 ml
  1 tsp. = 5 ml
  ½ tsp. = 2.5 ml
  I advise using standard kitchen measuring spoons for all recipes that require teaspoon or tablespoon amounts, and for doses.

- Adult doses are provided as standard for all remedies; children take the smaller end of the dose range, or ¼–½ the adult dose, unless otherwise specified. See page 94 for more details on doses, and see the box on page 24, "Taking Herbal Remedies."

Taking Herbal Remedies

*Herbal remedies can work remarkably well,
and sometimes they work fast. Often they are not a
quick fix, however, needing instead to be taken over
weeks and months to achieve the desired effect.
Recipes for medicines depend on empirical, traditional
knowledge, some of which (but not all) is backed up by
modern scientific research.*

◇◇◇◇◇◇◇◇◇◇◇◇◇◇◇◇◇◇

*Responsibility for self-prescribing any of the
remedies in this book falls solely with the reader.*

◇◇◇◇◇◇◇◇◇◇◇◇◇◇◇◇◇◇

*If you are pregnant or breastfeeding,
have any serious or long-lasting health condition,
or if you are already taking medication, it is
especially important to first seek the advice
of a healthcare professional.*

◇◇◇◇◇◇◇◇◇◇◇◇◇◇◇◇◇◇

The Recipes

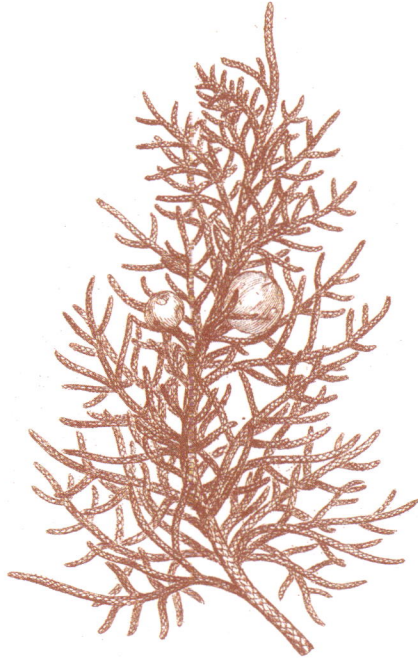

HOUSEHOLD PRODUCTS

The cleaners in this section are wonderful and effective environmentally friendly alternatives to strong-smelling chemicals. The essential oils leave a fresh clean smell and mildly disinfect the area. Herbs also make perfect room sprays and wonderful potpourri.

❦

Chamomile & Marjoram Surface Cleaner

The addition of chamomile and marjoram gives this gentle but effective eco-cleaner a beautiful, sweet scent.

INGREDIENTS
- 2 cups white distilled vinegar
- 2 tsp. marjoram flowers and leaves
- 1–2 tsp. chamomile flower heads
- 20 drops lavender essential oil

MAKES & KEEPS
Makes 2 cups.
Keeps up to 2 years.

METHOD
Make an infused vinegar with the herbs (p.19). Add the essential oil and decant into a spray bottle (for easy cleaning).

For everyday use, add an equal amount of water to the mixture. Spray on, wait for a few minutes, and wipe off.

For really tough jobs, use the cleaner undiluted; gently heating for a few minutes will make it extra strong. Spray dirty surfaces with hot vinegar cleaner and wait for 15 minutes before scrubbing and rinsing.

All-Purpose Cleaning Spray

Courtesy of Michael Vertolli

INGREDIENTS
- ¾ cup + 5 tsp. water, boiled or distilled
- 3 tbsp. + 1 tsp. white distilled vinegar
- 1 drop Liquid Castile Soap (p.199)

Essential oils:
- 5 drops lavender
- 3 drops pine
- 3 drops spruce or fir
- 1 drop geranium

MAKES & KEEPS
Makes 1 cup.
Keeps indefinitely.

METHOD
Combine the ingredients in a spray bottle and shake to mix.

Shake well before use. Spray the surface, then wipe clean.

Lemon-Fresh Cleaner

INGREDIENTS
- 2 cups white distilled vinegar
- I lemon, sliced

Essential oils:
- IO drops lemon
- IO drops orange

MAKES & KEEPS
Makes 2 cups.
Keeps I year or more.

METHOD
Make an infused vinegar with the lemon (p.19),
then add the essential oils.

Use as for Chamomile & Marjoram Surface
Cleaner (opposite).

Bug-Busting Surface Cleaner

INGREDIENTS
- 2 cups white distilled vinegar
- I–2 tsp. thyme leaves
- 2 tsp. marigold petals
- 20 drops thyme essential oil

MAKES & KEEPS
Makes 2 cups.
Keeps up to 2 years.

METHOD
Make an infused vinegar with the thyme and
marigold (p.19), then add the essential oil.

Use as for Chamomile & Marjoram Surface
Cleaner (opposite).

Anti-Bacterial Multisurface Cleaner

Courtesy of Teri Evans

INGREDIENTS
- I tsp. borax (see box, p.43)
- I tsp. baking soda
- 2 tsp. lemon juice
- I$\frac{2}{3}$ cups hot water

Essential oils:
- IO drops tea tree
- 5 drops eucalyptus
- 5 drops lavender

MAKES & KEEPS
Makes about I$\frac{2}{3}$ cups.
Keeps up to 2 months.

METHOD
Put all the ingredients into an empty spray
cleaner bottle. Shake well to mix, repeating
vigorously before each use.

Rinse surfaces after spraying to remove traces
of borax and oils.

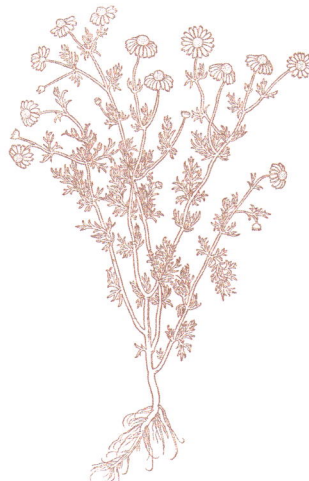

Zesty Dishwashing Liquid

INGREDIENTS
- 4 tsp. washing soda
- 1½ cups boiling water
- 5 tbsp. Liquid Castile Soap (p.199) or 1⅔ (4-oz.) bars solid castile soap, grated

Essential oils:
- 10 drops lemon or orange
- 10 drops grapefruit
- 10 drops tea tree

MAKES & KEEPS
Makes about 1¾ cups.
Keeps at least 6 months.

METHOD
If using grated soap, stir into the water until dissolved, then slowly stir in the soda. If not, dissolve the washing soda in the water, then add the liquid soap, continuing to stir until dissolved. Let cool. When cool, stir in the essential oils and bottle.

Shake well before use.

— *Tip* —

IF YOU USE GRATED
SOLID SOAP, YOUR HOMEMADE
DISHWASHING LIQUID MAY THICKEN
IN THE COLD. USING LESS WASHING
SODA WILL GIVE A THINNER LIQUID
IF YOU LIVE IN COLDER CLIMES.
ALWAYS RINSE WELL AFTER WASHING,
AS FOR ANY DISHWASHING LIQUID.

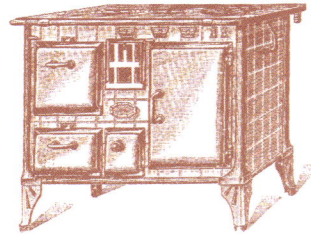

Eco-Powered Oven Cleaner with Basil

This is as effective as commercial brands, without the chemicals.

INGREDIENTS
- ½ cup Liquid Castile Soap (p.199)
- 1¼ cups baking soda
- ¼ cup rosemary vinegar (p.19)
- 4 drops basil essential oil (optional)

MAKES & KEEPS
Makes enough for one really thorough clean. Mix the cleaner up freshly each time you need it.

METHOD
Mix all the ingredients thoroughly in a bowl. Remove the oven shelves and clean separately.

Using a paintbrush, spread your mixture over the entire surface of the oven. Let it sit for 6–8 hours or overnight. During this time, the mixture will foam up slightly and lift the grime from the oven surface.

Using a bowl full of clean water and a damp foam scrubber, wipe out the oven. Change the water as needed. If the oven is really greasy and hasn't been cleaned for a while, repeat the process once again.

Rosemary & Pine Toilet Cleaner

INGREDIENTS
- 1 small handful of rosemary leaves
- 1 large handful of pine needles, removed from the stems
- 2 cups white distilled vinegar or Apple Cider Vinegar (p.165)
- 50 drops/½ tsp. rosemary essential oil (optional)
- 50 drops/½ tsp. pine essential oil (optional)

MAKES & KEEPS
Makes about 2 cups.
Keeps at least 1 year.

METHOD
Make an infused vinegar with the fresh rosemary and pine needles (p.19). If desired, add the essential oils for a stronger odor.

Pour a pail of water down the toilet to force water out of the bowl. This will enable you to reach the sides more easily. Then pour the undiluted cleaner into the bowl and let sit for 10–20 minutes. Scrub well with a toilet brush.

Thyme & Marigold Disinfectant

INGREDIENTS
- 2 cups white distilled vinegar or Apple Cider Vinegar (p.165)
- 100 drops/1 tsp. thyme essential oil
- ½ oz. dried thyme (or 1 handful of freshly picked, if possible, the leaves removed from the stems)
- ½ oz. dried marigold flowers (or 1 handful of fresh)

MAKES & KEEPS
Makes just under 2 cups.
Keeps at least 2 years.

METHOD
Make an infused vinegar with the thyme leaves and marigold flowers (p.19). Add the thyme essential oil and bottle the mixture.

Use it diluted 50:50 with water to wipe down surfaces, sinks, toilet seats, and pet areas.

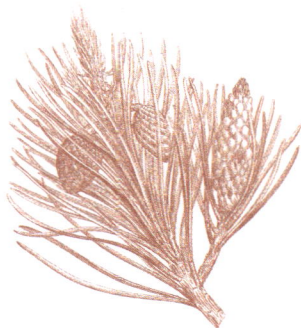

Lemon Zinger Floor Cleaner

Thyme & Marigold Disinfectant (p.29) forms the base of this floor cleaner, ideal for ceramic or vinyl tile floors. Do not use it on a stone floor, because vinegar can erode some types of stone, including marble.

INGREDIENTS
- 1 cup Thyme & Marigold Disinfectant (p.29)
- 3 cups white distilled vinegar
- ¾ cup lemon juice

MAKES & KEEPS
Makes enough for 4 washes. Keeps 3 months.

METHOD
Mix all the ingredients together.

Add 1¼ cups of the floor cleaner to a large pail (approx. 5 quarts) of hot tap water. Sweep the floor and clean with a mop (no need to rinse).

Stone Floor Soap

A little linseed in this stone floor cleaner adds extra shine.

INGREDIENTS
- 1 cup Liquid Castile Soap (p.199)
- 2 tbsp. linseed oil

Essential oils:
- 50 drops/½ tsp. grapefruit or orange
- 50 drops/½ tsp. tea tree
- just over ¾ cup hot water

MAKES & KEEPS
Makes just under 2 cups.
Keeps 3–6 months.

METHOD
Mix the liquid soap together with the linseed oil and essential oils. Pour the hot water over this mixture and stir gently.

To use, add 3 tbsp. to a large pail of hot water. Clean the floor thoroughly, using a mop. Rinse with clean water, if desired, but not essential.

Juniper, Rosemary & Lavender Glass Cleaner

INGREDIENTS
- 1 cup white distilled vinegar

Essential oils:
- 25 drops/¼ tsp. juniper
- 25 drops/¼ tsp. rosemary
- 25 drops/¼ tsp. lavender

MAKES & KEEPS
Makes 1 cup.
Keeps 1–2 years.

METHOD
Put the vinegar and oils into a spray bottle and shake gently. Let sit for 24 hours to settle.

To use, add 2 tsp. of the cleaner to 1 quart warm water. Do not use more than this, because it will lead to streaks.

Apply the diluted cleaner to the glass, using a clean cloth or spray from a bottle. Wipe the glass clean with a dry cloth.

— Tip —

TO AVOID STREAKS, DO NOT CLEAN WINDOWS WHEN THEY ARE WARM—EARLY MORNING OR DUSK IS THE BEST TIME.

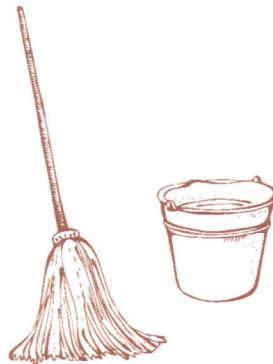

Rosemary & Horse Chestnut Scouring Powder

Baking soda lifts dirt off surfaces and is gently abrasive, so it can be used to make a scouring powder. Adding dried and powdered herbs brings abrasive qualities to the scouring mixture. The horse chestnuts also contain saponins, which have a detergent effect.

INGREDIENTS

- 4 dried horse chestnuts (the nuts only), ground
- ½ oz. dried rosemary leaves, ground
- 2 cups baking soda
- 2½ cups chickpea (besan) flour
- 20 drops rosemary essential oil (optional)

MAKES & KEEPS

Makes 5 cups.
Keeps 6–12 months.

METHOD

Put all the dry ingredients into a dry jar (if damp, the baking soda will react) with a tight-fitting lid. Shake well to mix. Sprinkle in the essential oil, if using, and mix again.

Sprinkle onto a damp cloth to clean bath rings, food deposits from the sink, etc. For a cream cleaner, mix a little powder with an equal amount of water to form a paste.

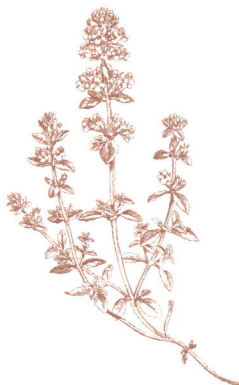

— Tip —

USE THE ROSEMARY & HORSE CHESTNUT SCOURING POWDER TO CLEAN STAINED TEA CUPS— IT'S MIRACULOUS.

Thyme Disinfectant Scouring Powder

INGREDIENTS

- 1 cup salt
- 15 drops thyme essential oil
- ½ oz. dried thyme leaves, ground
- 2 cups baking soda

MAKES & KEEPS

Makes 3¼ cups.
Keeps indefinitely.

METHOD

Spread the salt out on a plate and sprinkle thoroughly with the thyme oil. Mix all the ingredients together.

Use as for Rosemary & Horse Chestnut Scouring Powder (left).

Odor-Busting Natural Drain Cleaner

The herbs and baking soda control germs and help eliminate bad odors.

INGREDIENTS

- ½ oz. dried thyme leaves, ground
- ½ oz. dried rosemary leaves, ground

Essential oils:
- 50 drops/½ tsp. thyme
- 50 drops/½ tsp. basil
- 4 cups baking soda

MAKES & KEEPS

Makes about 4½ cups.
Keeps at least 1 year.

METHOD

Put the thyme and rosemary with the essential oils into a jar. Mix well. Add the baking soda, then shake and stir to mix thoroughly. Store in a dry, airtight jar.

To use, first run the hot tap water for a few minutes to warm up the drain. Then slowly pour about 1 teacup or half a mug of the scouring powder down the drain. Dribble in a little hot water to send it down the pipe. Let the cleaner work overnight, then rinse to clear.

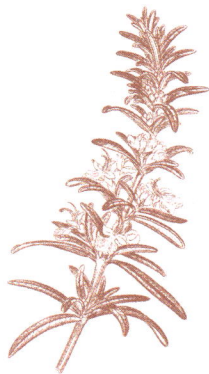

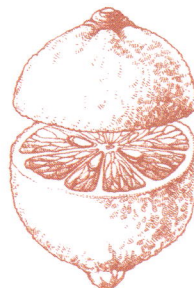

Lemon Furniture Polish

As well as nourishing the wood with oil and giving a great shine, this polish smells wonderful.

INGREDIENTS

- just over ¾ cup olive oil or linseed oil
- ¾ oz. dried lemon balm or lemongrass (or 1 large handful of fresh)
- ½ cup lemon juice (from about 4 lemons)

MAKES & KEEPS

Makes 1¼ cups.
Keeps 6–12 months.

METHOD

Make an infused oil with the oil and herbs (p.20). Mix the infused oil with the lemon juice and bottle.

Shake well before use. Rub well into wooden furniture or floors with a soft cloth. This mixture will also nourish your hands while you polish!

Spicy Furniture Polish

INGREDIENTS
- just over ¾ cup olive oil or linseed oil
- 2 tbsp. ground allspice
- just under ½ cup lemon juice, freshly squeezed or store-bought

MAKES & KEEPS
Makes 1¼ cups.
Keeps 6–12 months.

METHOD
Make an infused oil from the oil and mixed spice (p.20). Add the lemon juice to the mixture and bottle.

Use as for Lemon Furniture Polish (opposite).

— Tip —

USE SOFT COTTON CLOTHS FOR POLISHING, ONES THAT DON'T SHED THEIR FIBERS. I USE AN OLD COTTON SHEET CUT UP. MODERN MICROFIBER POLISHING CLOTHS ARE ALSO GOOD.

Old-Fashioned Furniture Polish

Courtesy of Teri Evans

This polish will improve your wood and should cut through residues left by spray polishes.

INGREDIENTS
- ½ cup turpentine or mineral spirits
- 1 cup + 1 tbsp. beeswax, grated or broken into small pieces
- 50 drops/½ tsp. lavender essential oil

MAKES & KEEPS
Makes about 1½ cups.
Keeps indefinitely.

METHOD
Gently heat the turpentine and beeswax together carefully in a double boiler or water bath. (Turpentine is flammable, so do not leave unattended.) When the wax is melted, pour into a jar and cool to lukewarm. Add the lavender essential oil and stir.

The lavender will release a lovely fragrance as you polish. It requires a little elbow grease, so you'll burn more calories using it!

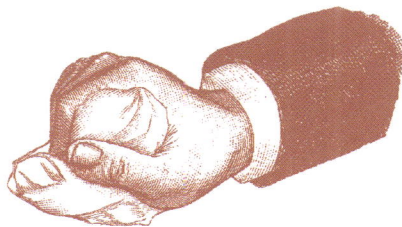

Plant-Based Wax for Raw Wood

INGREDIENTS

- I cup beeswax, grated or broken into small pieces
- I cup turpentine
- I cup boiled linseed oil
- 100 drops/I tsp. lavender essential oil

MAKES & KEEPS
Makes 3 cups.
Keeps 2 years.

METHOD
In a double boiler or water bath, melt the beeswax in the turpentine, then add the oil. In order to spread the wax easily it needs to be warm, so you may need to reheat the wax before using; return it to your double boiler if necessary.

Brush it warm onto raw wood (it sinks in). Work your way away from it, and when it has dried completely (30–60 minutes), buff it up into a shine with a soft cloth. The more you buff the wood, the shinier it gets. You can add layers to increase the shine.

Metal Polish

INGREDIENTS

- ¼ cup infused vinegar of your choice (p.19)
- ¼ cup fine clay powder or fine dirt from your own yard if you have that type where you live (avoid stone-filled or gritty soil, because it will scratch the metal)

MAKES & KEEPS
Makes ½ cup.
Keeps indefinitely.

METHOD
Mix the vinegar and dirt together in a bowl.

Rub the polish on your metal ornaments with a damp cloth. Wipe off with a dry soft polishing cloth and enjoy the shine. I have used this on brass, silver, and gold with good results.

— Variation —

THIS METAL POLISH CAN BE MADE WITH LEMON JUICE INSTEAD OF INFUSED VINEGAR, IF DESIRED, BUT WILL ONLY KEEP IN THE REFRIGERATOR FOR A WEEK.

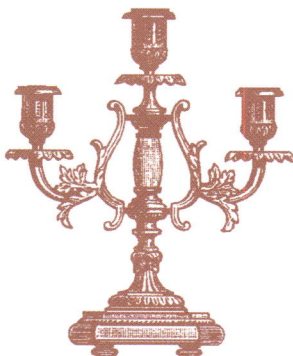

Citrus Carpet Cleaner

INGREDIENTS
Essential oils:
- 25 drops/¼ tsp. lemon
- 25 drops/¼ tsp. orange
- 25 drops/¼ tsp. lemongrass

- 2 cups white distilled vinegar
- Baking soda, as required

MAKES & KEEPS
Makes 2 cups.
Keeps indefinitely.

METHOD
Add the essential oils to the vinegar and mix well. Let sit for a day before use.

To treat stains, make a paste with a little of the vinegar and a small amount of baking soda. Shake before use. Brush well into the stained area (an old toothbrush is ideal for this job). Let it dry, then vacuum up.

You can also use this carpet cleaner diluted 1 part cleaner to 5 parts water in a carpet shampooing machine and 50:50 in a steam cleaner. Always check the manufacturer's instructions before using with your carpet shampooing machine or steam cleaner.

Spicy Laminate & Wooden Floor Cleaner

INGREDIENTS
- 1 cup white distilled or apple cider vinegar
- 2 cinnamon sticks, broken into pieces (or ½ oz. ground cinnamon)
- ¾ cup rubbing alcohol
- 2 tbsp. Liquid Castile Soap (p.199)
- 2 cups warm water
- 50 drops/½ tsp. orange essential oil

MAKES & KEEPS
Makes about 1 quart.
Keeps at least 1 year.

METHOD
Make an infused vinegar with the cinnamon sticks or ground cinnamon (p.19). Add the rubbing alcohol, liquid soap, warm water, and essential oil. Mix well and decant into a spray bottle for use.

Spray on and mop off with water.

Antibacterial Laminate & Wooden Floor Cleaner

INGREDIENTS
- 1 cup white distilled or apple cider vinegar
- ⅛ oz. marigold petals
- ¾ cup rubbing alcohol
- 2 tbsp. Liquid Castile Soap (p.199)
- 2 cups warm water
- 50 drops/½ tsp. thyme essential oil

MAKES & KEEPS
Makes about 1 quart.
Keeps at least 1 year.

METHOD
Make an infused vinegar with the marigold petals (p.19). Add the rubbing alcohol, liquid soap, warm water, and essential oil. Mix well.

Use as for Spicy Laminate & Wooden Floor Cleaner (left).

ROOM SPRAYS

Plant-based room sprays are widely used to freshen rooms. They play an important part in "space-clearing" or "energy-changing" exercises in the home. To make the sprays, put the ingredients into a 4-oz. spray bottle. Shake 24 times (a traditional number in feng shui) to make sure the essential oils are mixed, then spray abundantly around the room. It can be fun to add a small, specially programmed crystal to the bottle. All sprays, except the Fly Repellent on page 36, make just under ½ cup and keep for up to 3 months.

All these room sprays are courtesy of Lucy Harmer.

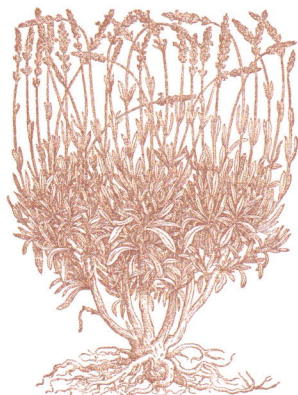

Happy House Air Spray

A rich scent used to bring happiness and fun into a home, and help to relieve depression.

INGREDIENTS
- **just under ½ cup spring water**

Essential oils:
- **12 drops basil**
- **12 drops orange**

Space-Clearing Spray

This refreshing and clean odor is said to clear "heavy" energy in the home.

INGREDIENTS
- **just under ½ cup spring water**

Essential oils:
- **14 drops juniper**
- **14 drops lavender**
- **14 drops rosemary**

Computer Energy Booster Spray

The effect of these clear-smelling oils increases concentration and boosts energy when you are working on a computer.

INGREDIENTS
- **just under ½ cup spring water**

Essential oils:
- **8 drops lemon**
- **8 drops lemongrass**
- **8 drops pine**

Helpful Angels Spray

Use when you are in need of divine assistance.

INGREDIENTS
- just under ½ cup spring water

Essential oils:
- 8 drops frankincense
- 8 drops myrrh
- 8 drops sandalwood

Emotional Balancing Spray

For when life's ups and downs are getting to you.

INGREDIENTS
- just under ½ cup spring water

Essential oils:
- 8 drops geranium
- 8 drops neroli
- 8 drops bergamot

Passion Spray

Speaks for itself!

INGREDIENTS
- just under ½ cup spring water

Essential oils:
- 8 drops ylang ylang
- 8 drops patchouli
- 8 drops amber

Love Spray

To encourage love of all types into your life.

INGREDIENTS
- just under ½ cup spring water

Essential oils:
- 8 drops rose
- 8 drops jasmine
- 8 drops sandalwood

Deep Sleep Spray

Zzzzzzzzzz!

INGREDIENTS
- just under ½ cup spring water

Essential oils:
- 12 drops lavender
- 6 drops chamomile
- 6 drops marjoram

Calm & Relaxation Spray

Destress with this lovely spray.

INGREDIENTS
- just under ½ cup spring water

Essential oils:
- 8 drops honeysuckle
- 8 drops cedar
- 8 drops vetivert

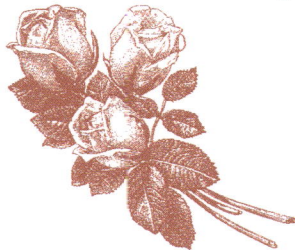

Protection Spray

These plants were traditionally used to protect the home against attacks or evil.

INGREDIENTS

- **just under ½ cup spring water**

Essential oils:
- **14 drops geranium**
- **14 drops sage**
- **14 drops petitgrain**

Prosperity Spray

This spray contains oils traditionally used to attract wealth.

INGREDIENTS

- **just under ½ cup spring water**

Essential oils:
- **6 drops mint**
- **6 drops cinnamon**
- **9 drops vetivert**
- **3 drops clove**

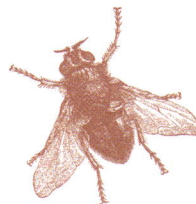

Fly Repellent

Courtesy of Teri Evans

This is a particularly strong mix to spray around doors and windows to repel flies and other insects. It is not for the body.

INGREDIENTS

- **¼ cup spring water**

Essential oils:
- **20 drops citronella**
- **20 drops lavender**

MAKES & KEEPS

Makes ¼ cup.
Keeps 3 months.

METHOD

Mix the water and essential oils together in the spray bottle.

Shake well, then spray around the window frames and doorframes. Avoid contact with skin and eyes, because this is a strong mix.

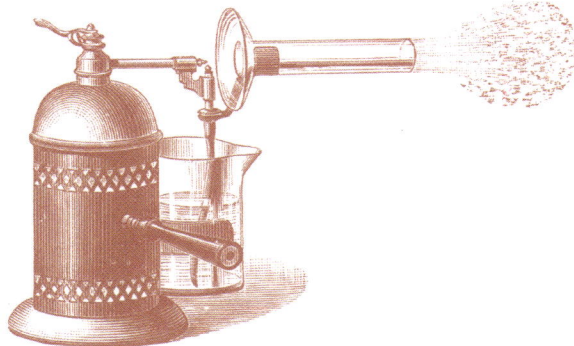

POTPOURRI

Potpourri is a collection of dried or semi-dried herbs, flowers, woods, and spices that is pleasant to the eye and gives off a lovely fragrance. Adding essential oils creates a stronger scent, and is also useful for refreshing the potpourri's fragrance.

To make any of these potpourris, mix together the dried plant materials in a beautiful bowl for display. Sprinkle the essential oils over the mix.

Each potpourri will keep well for 3–6 months. Refresh your mixture every so often with a few drops of essential oils.

> In our house, we are devotees of Radha and Krishna (the Divine Couple of the Vedic tradition), and almost every day we offer flowers on our altar to Thakurji (the Divine in statue form). I make potpourri from these special prasaadam flowers. *Prasaadam* means "mercy of God"; it gives you mercy or grace in the form of spiritual blessings.

Rainbow Potpourri

INGREDIENTS

- 2 handfuls of dried rose petals (red, pink, yellow, and orange)

A few of any of the following dried flowers and leaves:
- marigolds
- lavender
- hydrangea
- forget-me-nots
- lemon balm
- rosemary
- sage

Essential oils:
- 8 drops lavender
- 8 drops lemon balm
- 8 drops geranium
- 8 drops rose or rose geranium

Winter Festivities Potpourri

Collect together enough of the following to fill your chosen display bowl:

INGREDIENTS

- holly leaves (handle with care)
- holly berries
- cedar leaves
- ivy leaves
- small pinecones
- pine needles
- dried orange peel
- 1 tsp. cloves
- 1 nutmeg, freshly ground
- glitter, to add some sparkle (optional)

Essential oils:
- 10–20 drops cinnamon
- 10–20 drops orange
- 5–10 drops pine

Breathe-Easy Potpourri

This potpourri can help with breathing difficulties. Gather a mixture of the following to fill your bowl.

INGREDIENTS

- pine needles
- rosemary sprigs (broken into small pieces)
- eucalyptus leaves
- sage leaves
- bay leaves
- cedar leaves
- a few whole star anise

Essential oils:
- 10–20 drops peppermint
- 10–20 drops clary sage
- 10–20 drops pine

ECO-LAUNDRY PRODUCTS

Using eco-laundry products involves cleaning with a mixture of soap and alkaline substances (such as baking soda and washing soda), then removing soap residues and neutralizing the alkaline with vinegar. Herbs and oils are added for aroma and antimicrobial or soothing properties.

You can buy in solid and liquid soap to use in these recipes, or make your own. Soap making is fun and rewarding, but must be approached with care because it can be dangerous if not properly done. See page 194 for general instructions on soap making and molds, paying special attention to the safety measures.

Travelers' Antibug Laundry Soap

Courtesy of Tanya Smart

This variation gives travelers extra protection from bugs and insects.

INGREDIENTS

Lye:
- 5 oz. sodium hydroxide
- 14 oz. water

Oil blend:
- 4¾ oz. olive oil
- 6⅓ oz. sunflower oil
- 22 oz. coconut oil

Essential oils:
- 2½ tsp. lavender
- 100 drops/1 tsp. Virginian cedarwood
- 100 drops/1 tsp. juniper
- 50 drops/½ tsp. basil

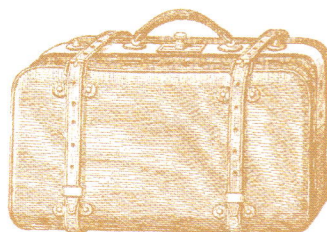

MAKES & KEEPS

Makes about 12–14 small bars (about 4 oz). Keeps years if well made, although the odor of the essential oils wears off.

METHOD

Follow the instructions as for Lavender Laundry Soap (opposite), taking note of the safety measures in the general soap-making instructions (p.194). First prepare the lye, then heat and cool the oils before adding the lye to them. Add the essential oils only after you have achieved "trace."

Lavender Laundry Soap

Courtesy of Tanya Smart

Handy for hand washing, stain removal, and a traveling laundry solution, this soap is used grated in laundry liquid and powder recipes.

INGREDIENTS

Lye:
- 5 oz. sodium hydroxide
- 14 oz. water

Oil blend:
- 4¾ oz. olive oil
- 6⅓ oz. sunflower oil
- 22 oz. coconut oil

Extras:
- 5 tsp. lavender essential oil

MAKES & KEEPS

Makes 12–14 small bars (about 4 oz.). Keeps several years.

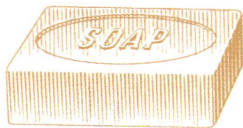

METHOD

Take note of the safety measures in the general soap-making instructions (p.194) before preparing this recipe.

Wearing gloves and plastic goggles, make the lye by carefully pouring the sodium hydroxide crystals into the container holding the water. Let it cool to 80–86°F. Never pour water onto the lye.

Gently heat the oil blend together until the coconut oil is melted, and cool until 80–86°F.

Carefully pour the lye into the oils and stir with the spatula until you reach "trace"; this is when the movement of the spatula creates a line on the top of the mixture—a trace that doesn't disappear. It is a sign that your soap has reached full saponification—when the lye has turned the oils to soap—and indicates your mixture is ready. To reach trace usually takes about half an hour, but soap has its own timescale! Keep stirring continuously and very thoroughly, all around the sides and the bottom of the pan.

When you've achieved a trace, add the essential oil. Ladle a little of the soap mixture into a bowl. Mix the essential oil into this small amount of soap mixture. Then mix this well into the whole batch.

Next, pour the mixture into mold(s) and cover (with a piece of board and then towels to insulate). Place the mixture out of the way for 24 hours.

After 24 hours, remove it from the mold(s), wearing gloves to protect against residual lye. Let sit for another 24 hours to dry. You can then cut up the soap if you need to.

Wash all your equipment with very hot water and plenty of dishwashing liquid. Wear dishwashing gloves (remember that the remnants will still be caustic) and rinse very thoroughly.

As with all soap, let it "cure" in a well-ventilated place for 4–6 weeks. This allows for all the caustic effect of the lye to wear off.

LAUNDRY LIQUIDS

To make these laundry liquids, first stir the washing soda into a little of the hot water in a pail until it is dissolved. Then add the baking soda (or borax, if using; see box opposite) and stir until dissolved. Mix in the liquid soap and stir gently to avoid too much frothing up.

When all of these ingredients are dissolved, add the essential oils and the rest of the water. Stir gently, then funnel into storage bottles. If you don't have liquid soap, you can add ¾–1 cup pure vegetable soap flakes or about half a bar of grated soap instead, dissolving it in a little boiling water before mixing in.

Shake well to remix before each use, or the ingredients will separate while standing.

For all these laundry liquids, with the exception of the Gentle Soap Nut Laundry Liquid on page 44, add ¼–⅓ cup per load of washing to the compartment or drum.

Citrus Laundry Liquid

INGREDIENTS
- ½–1 cup Liquid Castile Soap (p.199)
- 1 cup washing soda
- 1 cup baking soda or borax (borax makes a stronger mix, but baking soda is better for people with sensitive skin; see box, opposite)
- 4¾ quarts hot water

Essential oils:
- 100 drops/1 tsp. lemon
- 50 drops/½ tsp. grapefruit

MAKES & KEEPS
Makes 4¾ quarts.
Keeps at least 1 year.

Concentrated Lavender Laundry Liquid

INGREDIENTS
- ½–1 cup Liquid Castile Soap (p.199)
- 1 cup washing soda
- 1 cup baking soda or borax (borax makes a stronger mix, but baking soda is better for people with sensitive skin; see box, opposite)
- 4¾ quarts hot water
- 2 tsp. lavender essential oil

MAKES & KEEPS
Makes 4¾ quarts.
Keeps at least 1 year.

METHOD
Mix gently before each use. Use ¼–⅓ cup per load of washing.

— Tip —

ADD MORE LIQUID SOAP IF YOU NEED A STRONGER WASHING LIQUID. LIQUID CASTILE SOAP IS PREFERABLE, BUT IF YOU'RE UNABLE TO USE CASTILE, ANY LIQUID SOAP WILL DO.

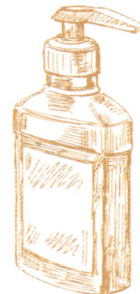

Spicy Laundry Liquid

INGREDIENTS
- ½–1 cup Liquid Castile Soap (p.199)
- 1 cup washing soda
- 1 cup baking soda or borax (borax makes a stronger mix, but baking soda is better for people with sensitive skin; see box, right)
- 4¾ quarts hot water

Essential oils:
- 100 drops/1 tsp. lavender
- 50 drops/½ tsp. orange
- 25 drops/¼ tsp. cinnamon

MAKES & KEEPS
Makes 4¾ quarts.
Keeps at least 1 year.

Luxury Laundry Liquid

INGREDIENTS
- ½–1 cup Liquid Castile Soap (p.199)
- 1 cup washing soda
- 1 cup baking soda or borax (borax makes a stronger mix, but baking soda is better for people with sensitive skin; see box, right)
- 4¾ quarts hot water

Essential oils:
- 100 drops/1 tsp. rose geranium
- 25 drops/¼ tsp. neroli
- 25 drops/¼ tsp. jasmine
- 10 drops rose (optional, as expensive!)

MAKES & KEEPS
Makes 4¾ quarts.
Keeps at least 1 year.

Antipsoriasis Laundry Liquid

INGREDIENTS
- ½ cup Liquid Castile Soap (p.199)
- 1 cup washing soda
- 1 cup baking soda
- 4¾ quarts hot water

Essential oils:
- 100 drops/1 tsp. lavender
- 50 drops/½ tsp. bergamot

MAKES & KEEPS
Makes 4¾ quarts.
Keeps at least 1 year.

Caution

Borax, or sodium borate, is a naturally occurring mineral salt found in dry lake beds. It is a strong cleanser and whitener, and can treat mildew. Borax contains boron, a chemical that occurs in all vegetables and fruits not grown on exhausted soil, and is important for brain, bone, and immune function. However, people with delicate, sensitive skin often find borax an irritant, and there is some evidence that it could be harmful to health, especially hormonal health, and the male reproductive system.

Borax substitutes can be made from washing soda mixed with soap and vinegar, but baking soda also works in the recipes. After researching this subject, I am happy to include borax in a recipe, but do research the subject yourself before making a decision. If you do use borax, as with any strong alkaloid, handle it with care; it can irritate the skin and should not be inhaled.

Gentle Soap Nut Laundry Liquid

This liquid is suitable for babies and young children, wool, and delicate fabrics.

INGREDIENTS
- ½ cup weak chamomile vinegar (made with 1 tsp. chamomile flowers infused in ½ cup white distilled vinegar for 1 week, p.19)
- 1 cup soap nuts
- 1 quart filtered or spring water

Essential oils (optional):
- 30 drops/⅓ tsp. lavender
- 30 drops/⅓ tsp. chamomile

MAKES & KEEPS
Makes around 2½ cups (enough for 20 loads in a washing machine).
Keeps 6–12 months.

METHOD
Put the vinegar, soap nuts, and water into a large, lidded pan. Place on medium heat and bring to a low boil. Simmer gently for 30 minutes with the lid on.

Remove from heat, mash the nuts (with a potato masher), and simmer for another 30 minutes, this time with the lid off to let the liquid reduce. Remove from heat.

When cool, strain the liquid and press well before adding the essential oils, if using. Store in an airtight container.

To use, add about ¼ cup per wash to your washing machine (half this in a high-efficiency machine). As with all washing liquids, you can put it in the drawer of the machine or in the drum.

Pets' Bedding Laundry Liquid

Use this to discourage fleas.

INGREDIENTS
- 1 cup Liquid Castile Soap (p.199)
- 1 cup washing soda
- 1 cup baking soda or borax (borax makes a stronger mix, but baking soda is better for people with sensitive skin; see box, p.43)
- 4¾ quarts hot water

Essential oils:
- 100 drops/1 tsp. lavender
- 50 drops/½ tsp. tea tree

MAKES & KEEPS
Makes 4¾ quarts.
Keeps at least 1 year.

METHOD
Mix gently before each use. Use ¼–⅓ cup per load of washing.

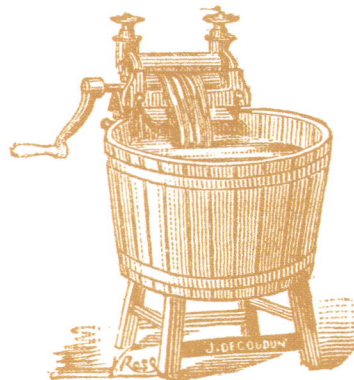

Space Clearer's Washing Powder

The essential oils in this recipe are used to cleanse and transform negative energy, so this powder is ideal for washing clothes before a space-clearing exercise.

INGREDIENTS

- 1 (3½–4-oz.) bar of laundry soap, grated (about 1 cup)
- ½ cup washing soda
- just over ¾ cup borax (see box, p.43); or use another ½ cup washing soda
- ½ cup baking soda

Essential oils:

- 50 drops/½ tsp. lavender
- 50 drops/½ tsp. rosemary
- 50 drops/½ tsp. juniper

YOU WILL NEED

· A FOOD PROCESSOR

MAKES & KEEPS

Makes enough for 30–60 washes.
Keeps 6 months or more.

METHOD

Make using the method for Superstrong Citrus Washing Powder (right). Use 1–2 tbsp. per wash.

— Tip —

BEFORE YOU USE THESE LAUNDRY POWDERS, DO ONE WASH WITH JUST A HALF MUG OF PLAIN WASHING SODA. THIS WILL CLEAN OUT ANY RESIDUES FROM YOUR OLD WASHING POWDER, WHICH COULD OTHERWISE REACT WITH YOUR HOMEMADE ECO-MIX AND CAUSE A YELLOW COLOR.

Superstrong Citrus Washing Powder

This recipe contains borax (see box, p.43), which must be handled very carefully.

INGREDIENTS

- 1 (3½–4-oz.) bar of laundry soap, grated (about 1 cup)
- ½ cup washing soda
- just over ¾ cup borax (see box, p.43); or use another ½ cup washing soda
- ½ cup baking soda

Essential oils:

- 50 drops/½ tsp. lemon
- 50 drops/½ tsp. mandarin or orange

YOU WILL NEED

· A FOOD PROCESSOR

MAKES & KEEPS

Makes enough for 30–60 washes.
Keeps 6 months or more.

METHOD

Add the essential oils to the soap, then whisk or mix in a food processor to make a finer, powdered soap.

Add the washing soda, borax, and baking soda to the food processor, and mix all the ingredients well for 3–5 minutes.

To use, add 1–2 tbsp. to the powder section of your washing machine drawer.

Baby Soft Washing Powder

INGREDIENTS

- I cup white distilled vinegar
- I tsp. chamomile flowers
- I tsp. rose petals
- I tsp. lavender flowers
- I cup finely grated Lavender Laundry Soap (p.41) or other vegetable oil soap
- I cup washing soda
- I cup baking soda

YOU WILL NEED
· A FOOD PROCESSOR

MAKES & KEEPS
Makes about 4 cups.
Keeps indefinitely in a sealed container.

METHOD
Make an infused vinegar of chamomile, rose, and lavender (p.19).

Put the grated soap into a large bowl. Stir in the washing soda and baking soda. Gradually pour in the infused vinegar, a little at a time. This will make it foam up and thicken into a paste, so don't add too quickly.

Whisk the mixture. You can do this by hand, but a food processor will be much easier, because it needs to be thoroughly mixed. Whisk until it becomes a powder, then let it sit for an hour. The mixture will appear even more powdery, just like a washing powder.

Stir again and store in a sealed (airtight) container. You will need 2–3 tbsp. for each full load of washing.

Soapwort Wool Wash

INGREDIENTS

- 2 oz. dried soapwort leaves and stems, or roots (or 3 cups of fresh)
- I quart water
- I cup white distilled vinegar (or floral vinegar as for Baby Soft Washing Powder, left)
- 20 drops lavender or lemon essential oil (optional)

YOU WILL NEED
· A FOOD PROCESSOR

MAKES & KEEPS
Makes about 2 cups "soapwort tea,"
enough for 3–4 washes.
Keeps 12 months.

METHOD
Boil the soapwort leaves and stems in the water for about 10 minutes (if you are using roots, boil for 20 minutes) with the lid on until the mixture has reduced by one-third. Let cool, then mix in a blender (the liquid will become frothy). Let sit for a few hours for the froth to die down, then strain well.

Add the white distilled vinegar, or the floral vinegar if you prefer a softer scent. Mix in the essential oil, if desired.

Store in an airtight container. To use, add ½–¾ cup to your washing water.

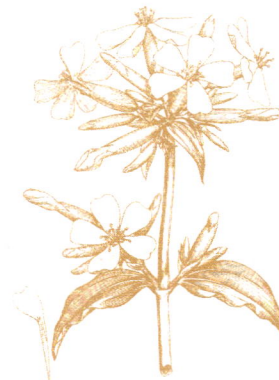

Zesty Stain Remover

The basic principle of a stain remover is to use a concentrated amount of washing product. Try using this on colorfast clothes.

INGREDIENTS
- ¼ cup Superstrong Citrus Washing Powder (p.45) or Baby Soft Washing Powder (opposite)
- juice of 1 lemon

MAKES & KEEPS
Makes about ¼ cup.
Keeps 2–3 months.

METHOD
Mix 1–2 tbsp. of your homemade washing powder with the lemon juice to make a paste. Then mix in the remaining washing powder. Store in a small jar.

As soon as you notice a stain, rub in a little of your stain-busting paste and put the item in the laundry basket to await its normal wash. As with all stain removers, this remover is most effective if you treat the stain before it sets.

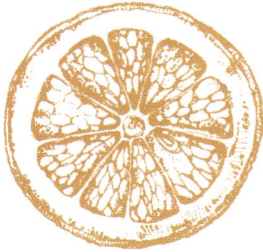

Eco-Powered Laundry Whitener

This fresh-smelling whitener relies on the bleaching power of lemon juice.

INGREDIENTS
- juice of 5 lemons
- 1 quart white distilled vinegar
- 20 drops lemon essential oil

MAKES & KEEPS
Makes about 1 quart (enough for 4–8 washes).
Keeps up to 6 months.

METHOD
Mix the ingredients together.

Add ½ cup of this whitener plus ¼–½ cup baking soda to your regular washing liquid/powder, plus another ¼–½ cup in the rinse compartment.

— *Tip* —

ANOTHER STAIN-REMOVAL METHOD
IS TO SCRUB UNDILUTED LIQUID CASTILE
SOAP (P.199) INTO STAINS. LET SIT FOR
30–60 MINUTES AND WASH AS NORMAL.

— *Tip* —

DRYING CLOTHES ON A CLOTHESLINE IN
THE SUN IS THE BEST WAY TO KEEP
CLOTHES FRESH, AND THE SUN ITSELF
IS THE BEST WHITENER.

Wood Ash Detergent-Free Washing Liquid

Courtesy of Marc Luyckx

Able to wash effectively in washing machines without any detergent, this is a very strong alkaline product (potash or lye). Prepare it on a tiled floor and wear gloves and goggles while working with it.

INGREDIENTS
- just over ½ pail of sifted wood ash
- boiling water

YOU WILL NEED
· A COFFEE FILTER

MAKES & KEEPS
Makes about ¼ pail.
Keeps indefinitely.

METHOD
Pour boiling water into the pail until it reaches 1½–2 inches above the ash. Mix it thoroughly, cover, and let sit for 12 hours, stirring occasionally.

Stir, then filter through a piece of cheesecloth. Carefully dispose of the ash (it is strongly alkaline) and rinse out the cloth and pail.

Let the liquid settle, then place a sheet of paper towel, folded into four, over the hole in a funnel. Add a coffee filter and strain the liquid through this into a solid plastic container. The liquid will be yellow to light brown, but it will not affect clothes in any way. (Note: There will be no suds.)

To use, put ½ cup of the washing product into the washing compartment of your machine. Add ½ cup vinegar-base fabric softener (opposite) into the washing compartment. Note: For washes at 32–86°F, use half as much again of both liquid and of vinegar.

For whitening: Add an equal volume of washing soda with hot water and the washing liquid to the washing compartment.

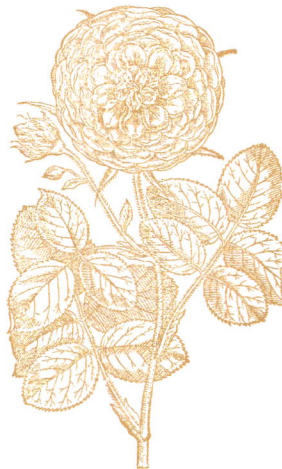

SOFT-TOUCH HERBAL FABRIC CONDITIONERS

These easy-to-make fabric conditioners use a weak infused vinegar as their base. Vinegar, an acid, basically removes all traces of soap from the fabric, making it feel soft.

All these recipes make 1 quart (enough for about 12 washes).

Sweet & Soft Fabric Conditioner with Rose

INGREDIENTS
- 1 tbsp. fragrant rosebuds or petals
- 1 quart white distilled vinegar

Essential oils:
- 50 drops/½ tsp. lavender
- 25 drops/¼ tsp. chamomile
- a few drops rose essential oil (optional)

KEEPS
Keeps 1–2 years.

METHOD
Infuse the roses in the vinegar (p.19). Add the essential oils to the infused vinegar.

To use, put ⅓ cup into the rinse compartment of the washing machine.

Skin-Calm Fabric Softener

INGREDIENTS
- 2 tbsp. marigold flowers
- 1 quart white distilled vinegar

Essential oils:
- 50 drops/½ tsp. lavender
- 50 drops/½ tsp. bergamot
- a few drops rose essential oil (optional)

KEEPS
Keeps 1–2 years.

METHOD
Infuse the marigold flowers in the vinegar (p.19). Then add the essential oils to the infused vinegar.

To use, put ⅓ cup into the rinse compartment of the washing machine.

Antibacterial Fabric Softener

INGREDIENTS
- 1 quart white distilled vinegar

Essential oils:
- 50 drops/½ tsp. lavender
- 50 drops/½ tsp. tea tree
- 25 drops/¼ tsp. thyme

KEEPS
Keeps indefinitely.

METHOD
Mix all the ingredients together and bottle.

Use ½ cup in the rinse stage of your wash (check the manufacturer's instructions for how to do this in your machine).

Pets' Bedding Fabric Conditioner

INGREDIENTS
- 1 quart white distilled vinegar

Essential oils:
- 50 drops/½ tsp. lavender
- 50 drops/½ tsp. orange
- 50 drops/½ tsp. tea tree

KEEPS
Keeps indefinitely.

METHOD
Make and use as described for Antibacterial Fabric Softener (above).

HERBAL MOTH REPELLENTS

Traditional moth balls are toxic, so you might want to make your own plant-power alternatives.

To make each of the moth-repellent sachets, you will need a small piece of thin cotton cloth cut into a circle about 6 inches in diameter, as well as silk or wool thread. Simply mix the dried herbs together in a bowl and sprinkle the essential oil, if using, over the mixture. Then lay your cloth on a flat surface and spoon half your herb mixture into the center. Draw together the sides of the cloth and fasten tightly at the top with a piece of wool or silk thread.

Each of the moth-repellent recipes makes two sachets, which will keep well for up to a year.

Before you pack away clothes for storing, make sure they are properly cleaned. Use a fabric conditioner as a rinse after washing. Air clothes well in the sun if you can before packing, then place these moth-repellent sachets between your folded clothes.

Lavender & Rosemary Moth Repellent

INGREDIENTS
Dried herbs:
- **2 tsp. lavender flowers**
- **2 tsp. rosemary leaves and flowers**
- **I tsp. thyme leaves**
- **I tsp. cloves**

Cedar & Southernwood Moth Repellent

INGREDIENTS
Dried herbs:
- **2 tsp. cedar wood, ground into small shavings**
- **2 tsp. southernwood leaves**
- **I tsp. cloves**
- **I tsp. thyme leaves**

Essential oils (optional):
- **20 drops lavender**
- **20 drops cedarwood**

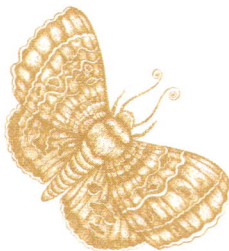

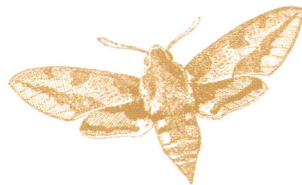

Moth-Destroying Spray

*If you already have moths, stronger methods
are needed.*

INGREDIENTS
- 1 quart boiling water
- 2 oz. dried thyme
- ¾ oz. dried cloves
- 2 tbsp. neem oil

Essential oils:
- 50 drops/½ tsp. thyme
- 50 drops/½ tsp. lemon

- 1 tsp. Liquid Castile Soap (p.199)

MAKES & KEEPS
Makes 1 quart.
Best used fresh, but will keep for 1–2 months.

METHOD
Pour the boiling water onto the thyme and
cloves. Let cool, then strain and add the neem
oil and essential oils, plus the liquid soap. Mix
thoroughly and store in a spray bottle.

If possible, put the affected clothes in the
freezer for 2 days to begin the moth-killing
process. Then spray them once, thoroughly,
with your moth-destroying spray. Check
carefully for signs of moths every week or so
for a few weeks following. Repeat the process,
if required.

Desert-Style Moth Repellent

INGREDIENTS
Dried herbs:
- 2 tsp. shredded sagebrush
- 2 tsp. white sage
- 1 tsp. cloves
- 1 tsp. southernwood

Essential oils (optional):
- 20 drops clove
- 20 drops sage

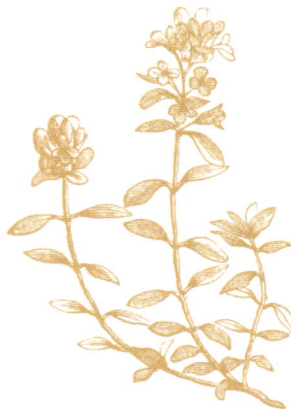

KEEPING WELL

Here you will find a range of do-it-yourself mineral and vitamin supplements, tonics, and teas that can be taken every day, as well as protection and nourishment for the skin, remedies for the mind and spirit, and more.

Flaxseed Rehydration Tea

Being fully hydrated can make an enormous difference to how well you feel, and remain. Tea from flaxseeds is perfect for rehydrating. Rich in omega-3 fatty acids from the seeds, the tea nourishes the cell membranes, and tones and protects the digestive tract from top to bottom. This recipe gives maximum rehydration.

INGREDIENTS
- **2 tbsp. flaxseeds**
- **I quart water**

MAKES & KEEPS
Makes about I cup, enough for 3 days. Keeps up to 3 days in the refrigerator.

METHOD
Put the seeds and water into a saucepan and bring to a boil. Remove from the heat and let sit with the lid on for 12 hours or overnight. The next day, bring to a boil again and simmer for I hour.

Strain the tea, reserving the seeds. (These can be eaten, for example, added to oatmeal or to a cookie dough, with some golden raisins.)

Put ¼ cup of the remaining liquid into a large (ideally 20-fl.-oz.) mug. Dilute the thick liquid with half boiling and half cold water. Drink I mug of the tea 3 times daily, half an hour before a meal.

— Tip —
IF YOU ARE IN A RUSH, YOU CAN MAKE FLAXSEED TEA THE QUICK WAY. THIS SIMPLE METHOD MAKES ENOUGH FOR ONE DAY'S TEA: BOIL I TBSP. OF FLAXSEEDS AND I CUP WATER IN A SAUCEPAN UNTIL THE WATER IS REDUCED BY HALF. DRINK ONCE OR TWICE DAILY TO SOOTHE IRRITATION. THE TEA KEEPS FOR UP TO 3 DAYS IN THE REFRIGERATOR.

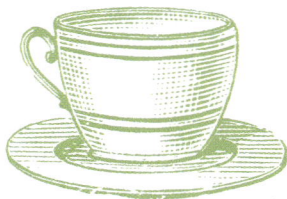

Probiotic Lemonade

Courtesy of Lynn Rawlinson

This delicious, probiotic drink can help restore the good bacteria in our digestive tract, easing bloating, irritable bowel syndrome (IBS), and trapped gas.

INGREDIENTS
- 1 (16-oz.) container probiotic plain organic yogurt (see below)
- ½ cup sugar
- ½ cup honey
- 3½–4 quarts freshly filtered water, to top up as required
- juice from 12 lemons

MAKES & KEEPS
Makes up to 4 quarts.
Keeps up to 2 weeks in the refrigerator.

METHOD
First make a whey: Put a thickish piece of cheesecloth over a bowl and attach it with a thick rubber band or string. Pour the yogurt into it and let sit for 1 hour.

Scoop the yogurt back into its container. In the bowl, you will have a clearish liquid—the whey containing the probiotics or helpful bacteria.

Place the sugar and honey into a large glass jar wth a lid. Add the whey and fill the jar halfway with fresh water. Add the lemon juice and top up again so that the jar is about three-quarters full. Tighten the lid. Mix the ingredients well by agitating the jar.

Keep at room temperature for 2 days; the probiotics in the whey will eat some of the sugar and multiply, leaving you with a probiotic lemonade ready to bottle.

— *Tip* —

THIS LEMONADE IS SHARP, SO YOU MAY
LIKE TO SWEETEN IT WITH HONEY
BEFORE DRINKING.

Soothing Sloe C Syrup

Courtesy of Rachel Corby

High in vitamin C, this syrup can help soothe bronchial conditions, colds, catarrh, and inflammation of the throat.

INGREDIENTS
- 1 cup fresh sloes (the fruit of blackthorn)
- 2 cups hot water
- 1½ cups honey

MAKES & KEEPS
Makes about 3 cups.
Keeps up to 2 years in the refrigerator.

METHOD
Decoct the sloes in the water (p.15) for 20 minutes. Do not boil. Strain and discard all the pits and plant matter.

Measure the remaining liquid. Either match what you have left with an equal volume of honey or discard any excess water so that only 1½ cups remain, then add the honey. Gently heat the liquid until all the honey has dissolved, and bottle.

Take 2 tsp. 3 times a day directly from a spoon or dissolved in an herbal tea.

Do not use if pregnant or breastfeeding.

— *Tip* —

IF POSSIBLE, COLLECT THE
SLOES AFTER A HARD FROST, BECAUSE
THIS MAKES THEIR SKIN SOFTER AND
MORE PERMEABLE. IF YOU WANT TO
MAKE THE SYRUP BEFORE THE FIRST
FROST, FREEZE THE SLOES BRIEFLY
BEFORE USING.

Rose Hip C Syrup

In Britain during World War II, there was a shortage of fruit, so vitamin C deficiency became a concern. The Women's Institute (WI) organized mass gatherings of rose hips and produced rose hip syrup on a large scale, made using a recipe provided by the Ministry of War. This recipe is based on that.

INGREDIENTS

- 4 cups fresh rose hips, finely chopped
- 3½ cups boiling water
- 2 cups cold water
- 1 cup sugar

YOU WILL NEED

- DOUBLE THICKNESS CHEESECLOTH OR JELLY BAG

MAKES & KEEPS

Makes about 2 cups.
Keeps for 1 year until opened, then keep in the refrigerator and use within 1 month.

METHOD

Drop the freshly picked and finely chopped rose hips into the boiling water. Stir, remove from the heat, and let sit for 20 minutes. Strain by letting it drip through the double thickness cheesecloth or the jelly bag. Transfer the hips from the cheesecloth to a saucepan. Wash the cheesecloth or jelly bag immediately after—you'll need it for the next stage of the recipe.

Add the strained juice and 2 cups of cold water to the pan. Bring to a boil. Stir, remove from heat, and let sit for 10 minutes. (Doing it twice ensures you get all the vitamin C.)

Strain again through the cheesecloth or jelly bag. Do not squeeze, but let it drip. This is to avoid tiny, irritating rose hip hairs getting into your preparation. As an extra precaution, pour back the first ½ cup of liquid that comes through, and make it drip through again.

Put the juice into a clean saucepan, bring to the boil, then boil with the lid off for 5 minutes. Add the sugar and boil briskly for another 5 minutes. Pour into small, sterilized jars.

Pour onto desserts and cereal, drink mixed with hot or cold water, or take 1–2 tsp. up to 3 times daily to protect against colds and flu.

— *Tip* —

TO FURTHER PRESERVE SYRUPS, STERILIZE THEM AFTER BOTTLING (SEE PP. 21–22).

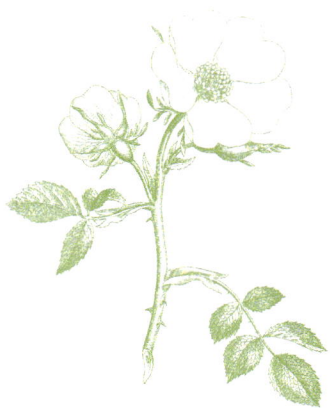

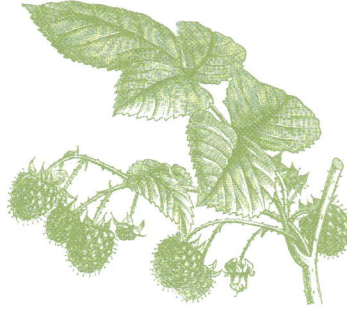

Many Berry Syrup

Courtesy of Wizz Holland

This syrup is delicious with carbonated water or poured over ice cream or yogurt. It is rich in vitamin C, so you can also take it like a medicine, a spoonful as it is or diluted in hot water, to ward off or treat colds.

INGREDIENTS

- 1 cup fresh berries (a mix of hawthorn, rose hips, elderberries, blackberries, raspberries, or whatever you can find)
- 2 cups water
- juice of 1–2 lemons
- 1½ cups honey

MAKES & KEEPS

Makes about 3 cups.
If unopened, will keep 1 year in the refrigerator. Once opened, drink within a few weeks.

METHOD

Make in the same way as Soothing Sloe Syrup (p.53), but add the lemon juice to each just over ¾ cup of liquid before adding the honey. Keep the pulp to make Many Berry Fruit Leather (p.56).

Elder, Rose Hip & Rowanberry Oxymel

This is a vitamin C–packed, immune–boosting honey and vinegar delight.

INGREDIENTS

2 handfuls of each of the following, removed from the stems:

- elderberries
- rose hips
- rowanberries
- 1 quart Apple Cider Vinegar (p.165)
- about 2¼ cups honey

MAKES & KEEPS

Makes about 5 cups.
Keeps around 2 years.

METHOD

Make an infused vinegar with the berries (p.19).

Measure the liquid and add an equal amount of honey. Gently heat to dissolve, then bottle.

Take 1–2 teaspoons 3–4 times daily to help fight viral infections.

Many Berry Fruit Leather

Courtesy of Wizz Holland

*This recipe was inspired by the lush-smelling pulp
leftovers from making Many Berry Syrup (p.55).*

INGREDIENTS
- 2–3 cups fruit pulp, leftovers from the
  Many Berry Syrup (p.55), plus what you
  need of apples, blackberries, rose hips,
  etc. to make up the volume
- juice of 1 lemon
- ½ cup honey

YOU WILL NEED
· FLAT BAKING SHEETS, LINED WITH WAX PAPER
· ADDITIONAL WAX PAPER, FOR ROLLING THE
  LEATHER

MAKES & KEEPS
Makes 20–30 strips.
Keeps 1–2 weeks, or up to 3 months if frozen.

METHOD
In a saucepan, gently cook the pulp with the
added fruits until all are mushy. Push the pulp
through a strainer to remove seeds, stems, and
so on, then mix in the lemon juice and honey.

Spread the mixture out thinly and fairly evenly
over the lined baking sheets. Let dry out in
an oven set on the lowest temperature for
3–5 hours, or until it feels rubbery but set.

Slice into strips and make little rolls. Do this
by rolling the strips together with a strip of
wax paper or aluminum foil, to avoid the
mixture sticking to itself. Store in a big jar,
ideally glass so that you can enjoy looking at
the colorful collection.

— Tip —

YOU CAN USE ANY FRUIT TO
MAKE "LEATHER" IN A SIMILAR WAY.
EXPERIMENT BY ADDING TASTY AND
FRAGRANT FLOWERS, SUCH AS ROSE
OR HONEYSUCKLE, OR SPICES.

Easy Iron Tonic

A very simple, easy-to-make iron and mineral tincture.

INGREDIENTS
- 1 cup unsulfured (brown) dried
  apricots (or hunza apricots, pitted),
  coarsely chopped
- 1 tbsp. molasses
- ½ oz. dried nettle tops (or 1 cup fresh),
  coarsely chopped
- 3 cups vodka

MAKES & KEEPS
Makes 3 cups. Keeps at least 2 years.

METHOD
See pp.18–19 for full instructions on how to
make tinctures.

Put all the ingredients into a jar, seal, and let sit
to brew. After 4 weeks, strain the liquid through
cheesecloth and bottle.

Take 2 tsp. daily in warm water or lightly
carbonated water as an iron tonic. If you are
anemic, support your liver by taking 1 tsp.
1–2 times daily of the tincture component of the
Detox Complex (p.61). Easy Iron Tonic is not
suitable for children under 7.

Supergreen Juice

*This juice is incredibly nutritious, packed with
minerals, vitamins, and health-giving enzymes.*

INGREDIENTS
- 2 oz. fresh wheatgrass or oat grass

YOU WILL NEED
· A JUICER

MAKES & KEEPS
Makes ¼ cup juice.
Drink immediately.

METHOD
Put the grass through a juicer and enjoy.
If you don't have a juicer, just add the grass
to a smoothie.

Vinegar Calcium Tonic

Courtesy of Jeanne Rose

An edible tincture for healthy bones, full of calcium.

INGREDIENTS
- **3 handfuls of fresh dandelion roots and leaves (dig these up yourself or buy them at a farmers' market), coarsely chopped**
- **about 2⅔ cups Apple Cider Vinegar (p.165)**

MAKES & KEEPS
Makes about 2 cups.
Keeps I year.

METHOD
Make an infused vinegar with the dandelion (p.19), letting it infuse for 6 weeks. The roots will develop and exude a milky substance into the vinegar.

Strain and bottle.

Use in salad dressings and marinades or sprinkled over cooked greens. Each tbsp. contains more than 175mg calcium—one-sixth of the adult recommended daily allowance.

Detoxing Mineral Vinegar

Nettles are a panacea of the plant world, used for aching joints, skin allergies, or a general detoxing/cleansing. They are rich in minerals, vitamins, and protein (p.241).

INGREDIENTS
- **3 handfuls of freshly picked nettle tops (or dried if you can't get fresh)**
- **2 cups Apple Cider Vinegar (p.165)**

MAKES & KEEPS
Makes 2 cups.
Keeps 2 years.

METHOD
Make an infused vinegar with the nettles (p.19).

Take I–2 tbsp. daily, in water or with food.

Leafu Protein Supplement

Courtesy of Michael Cole

There is a way of making "leafu," an edible curd, from grass and stinging nettles to access the valuable protein and amino acids they contain.

INGREDIENTS
- **2 lb. freshly picked nettle tops (mixed with any other edible greens, including grass, if desired)**

YOU WILL NEED
· A BLENDER

MAKES & KEEPS
Makes about I oz. leafu (enough for 2 meals).
Keeps up to I week in the refrigerator.

METHOD
Puree the nettles in a blender, adding a small amount of water, if necessary. Filter the juice through fine cloth.

Heat the filtered juice just up to boiling point, so that a green "froth" appears on the surface. Skim it off and put in a fine cloth (the holes need to be tiny to retain the "froth," which contains the protein). This "froth" can be eaten freshly as it is or added to smoothies, soups, or stews.

Alternatively, make into a curd by pressing slowly but firmly to get all the fluid out (this may take several hours). The protein-rich curd can be cut up and added to food.

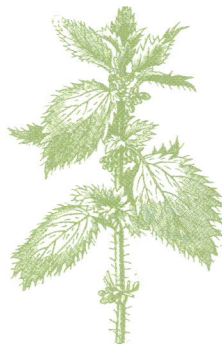

Multimineral Powder

Wild plants are often richer in minerals than cultivated ones. This wild herb powder can be sprinkled onto soups and stews or added to smoothies or juices for an instant health boost.

INGREDIENTS
Collect as many of the following wild herbs as you can:
- **burdock root**
- **dandelion leaves and root**
- **nettle leaves and root**
- **plantain leaves**
- **ground elder leaves**
- **peppermint**
- **red clover**
- **thyme**
- **sage**
- **yellow dock root**

Alternatively, buy a range of dried herbs.

KEEPS
I year.

METHOD
Dry the plant material and grind to a powder in a coffee grinder. Mix thoroughly and store in an airtight container.

Take 2–3 tsp. daily as a food supplement. You can add to a green smoothie or infuse in vinegar to make a multimineral vinegar (p.19).

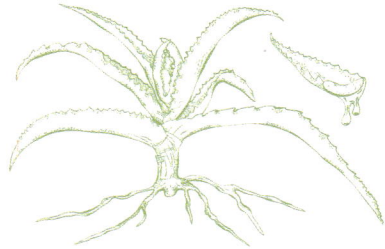

Aloe Vera Nourish All

Aloe vera contains hundreds of health-giving nutrients. To get the full benefit from this amazing miracle plant, use the leaves fresh.

INGREDIENTS
- **½ aloe vera leaf, without the green skin**
- **½ cucumber, chopped**
- **½ cup apple juice, freshly juiced or bought**

YOU WILL NEED
· A BLENDER

MAKES & KEEPS
Makes ⅔ cup.
Eat immediately.

METHOD
Cut the aloe vera leaf lengthwise and scrape out the gel inside. Add the gel to the other ingredients in a blender and blend until smooth.

Drink once a week, taking a month off every 6 months. Do not take continuously without a break.

Do not use aloe vera internally during menstruation, if you are pregnant, or if you have liver or gallbladder problems or hemorrhoids.

Milk Vetch, Ginseng & Nettle Stress Support Tonic

INGREDIENTS
- 2 oz. dried milk vetch root, chopped
- 2 oz. dried ginseng root, chopped
- 2 oz. dried Siberian ginseng root, chopped
- I quart water
- I cup chopped fresh nettle tops (or I oz. dried)
- 2 tbsp. good-quality honey (preferably manuka)
- 2 cups pure vegetable glycerin

MAKES & KEEPS
Makes I quart.
Keeps I year.

METHOD
Decoct the roots, boiling in the water for 15 minutes in a large, covered saucepan (p.15). Add the nettles and let cool.

Strain and, if necessary, boil further to reduce reduce it or add water to produce 2 cups of liquid. Remove from the heat and let cool for 10 minutes.

Add the honey and stir to dissolve. Add the glycerin and mix well, then bottle.

Take I tsp. 2–3 times daily to boost immunity and relieve stress.

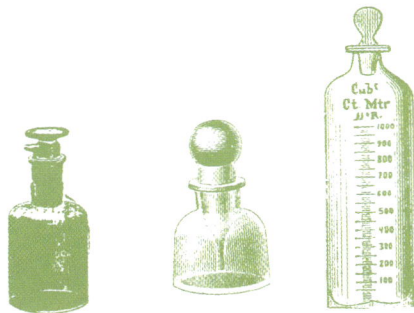

Walnut Flower Remedy for Adapting to Change

Courtesy of Lucy Harmer

Flower remedies harness flowers' energetic properties to help balance emotions. The most famous one is Dr. Bach's Rescue Remedy. Following tradition, make flower remedies on a bright sunny day around 10 a.m.

INGREDIENTS
- 3–4 stems of walnut flowers/leaves, about 6 inch in length (gather mainly female flowers; see box, below).
- 2 cups water
- about I cup brandy (more if required)

MAKES & KEEPS
Makes about 2 cups.
Keeps 2 years.

METHOD
Put the flowers and leaves into a saucepan with the water. Bring to a boil and simmer for about 30 minutes without a lid, stirring constantly. Remove from heat, add the lid. and let cool.

Strain into a glass bottle. Mix with an equal amount of brandy.

Keep in a dark place and fill a dropper bottle when you want to use.

Take 3–5 drops 3 times a day or when you are feeling stressed.

Female walnut flowers are small and green and have a figlike shape, while the male flowers are fat green catkins.

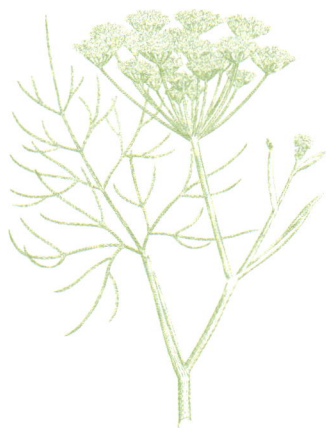

Weight Loss Spice

A spice mix of plants that help to burn fat.

INGREDIENTS
Dried herbs:
- 1 oz. ground ginger
- 1 oz. ground cardamom
- 1 oz. ground turmeric
- 5 tsp. cayenne pepper

MAKES & KEEPS
Makes about 3 oz.
Keeps 1 year.

METHOD
Mix the spices together well.

Drink as a tea, using 1 tsp. of spice per mug of boiling water (p.15). Drink 2–3 times daily.

Weight Loss Tea

These herbs can help to calm the appetite and speed metabolism without making you jumpy. Use alongside a healthy diet and also consider a detox program.

INGREDIENTS
- 2 oz. green tea
- 1 oz. fennel seeds
- 1 oz. dried dandelion leaves

MAKES & KEEPS
Makes 4 oz.
Keeps at least 1 year.

METHOD
Mix the ingredients together well. Make the tea using 1 tsp. per mug (p.15).

Drink 2–4 mugs daily.

— *Variation* —

ALTERNATIVELY,
MAKE A SOLID SPREAD.
TO DO THIS, MELT A 12-OZ. JAR
OF EXTRA-VIRGIN COCONUT OIL BY
PLACING THE JAR INTO A BOWL OF HOT
WATER. ONCE MELTED, MIX THE SPICES
IN THOROUGHLY. LET SET. TAKE 1 TSP.
2–3 TIMES DAILY EITHER DIRECTLY OFF
THE SPOON OR ADDED TO FOOD.
(ALTHOUGH IT IS AN OIL, COCONUT OIL
SPEEDS METABOLISM AND HELPS
THE BODY TO BURN OFF FAT.)

Detox Complex

Courtesy of Louise Idoux

In this mixture, the herbs encourage the liver to clear toxins into the bile. The prune juice takes them out of the body through bowel movements.

INGREDIENTS
Tinctures (either bought or homemade, pp.18–19) of the following:
- 2 tbsp./30ml milk thistle seeds
- 4 tsp./20ml dandelion root
- 5 tsp./25ml burdock root
- 5 tsp./25ml artichoke leaves

- just under ½ cup prune juice

MAKES & KEEPS
Makes just over ¾ cup.
Keeps up to 2 years.

METHOD
Mix the ingredients together and bottle.

Take 2 tsp. in a little water 3 times daily.

Do not give detoxing medicines to children under 12.

Detox Tea

This makes a mixture of dried herbs from which to make a daily tea.

INGREDIENTS
Dried herbs:
- ½ oz. nettle tops
- ½ oz. dandelion leaves
- ½ oz. ginger root, coarsely ground
- ½ oz. dandelion root, coarsely ground
- ½ oz. burdock root, coarsely ground
- 2 cinnamon sticks, coarsely ground

MAKES & KEEPS
Makes 3½ oz.
Keeps 1 year.

METHOD
Mix the ingredients and store in a jar.

Make tea using 1 tsp. per mug of boiling water. Let infuse for 5–10 minutes (p.15).

Drink 1–3 mugs daily, adding fresh lemon juice, and honey to taste.

Do not give detoxing medicines to children under 12. Detoxing of any kind is not recommended during pregnancy or breastfeeding. If you have any health problems, you should only undertake detoxing with the guidance of a qualified healthcare practitioner.

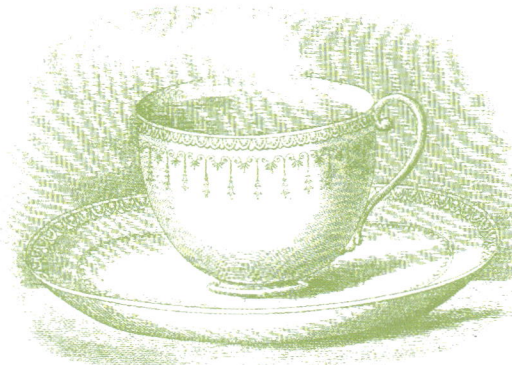

Mineral-Rich Seaweed Bath

To nourish the skin, encourage detoxification, relieve muscle and joint stiffness, and help the circulation.

INGREDIENTS
- 1 oz. dried kelp
- 1 oz. dried dulse

MAKES
Makes enough for 1 bath.

METHOD
It works best to put dried seaweed into a cheesecloth bag, otherwise it blocks your drain and is difficult to clean up. If you can gather fresh seaweed, put a couple of handfuls of each into your bathtub while running the water.

Soak in as hot a bath as is comfortable for around 30 minutes.

The Big Cleanser Smoothie

Courtesy of Neil McNulty

INGREDIENTS
- 1 apple
- 2 small bananas
- 2 handfuls of mixed fresh or frozen berries
- juice of 1 lemon (no seeds)
- 10 fresh rosemary leaves (no stems)
- Herbal tea: 1 small mug with peppermint (1 tsp. or 1 tea bag) and nettle (2 tsp. or 2 tea bags), infused for 5–10 minutes

YOU WILL NEED
· A BLENDER

MAKES & KEEPS
Makes 1–2 servings.
Drink immediately.

METHOD
Blend all the ingredients together and drink immediately.

Warm the Bones Smoothie

Courtesy of Neil McNulty

Ideal for people who feel the cold, or for treating rheumatism.

INGREDIENTS
- 1-inch piece fresh ginger root
- ½ tsp. ground cinnamon
- 1 tsp. ground turmeric
- 3 tbsp. coconut milk (or probiotic plain organic yogurt)
- 2 large bananas
- 2 pears
- Herbal tea: 1 small mug of chamomile tea (made from 1 tsp. dried chamomile or 1 tea bag infused for 5–10 minutes).

YOU WILL NEED
· A BLENDER

MAKES & KEEPS
Makes 1–2 servings. Drink immediately.

METHOD
Blend all the ingredients together and drink right away.

Winter Warmer Tea

INGREDIENTS
- ¾ oz. dried ginger root
- 2 cinnamon sticks
- ¾ oz. dried licorice root

MAKES & KEEPS
Makes 2-oz. herb mixture.
Keeps 1 year.

METHOD
Loosely grind the ginger, cinnamon, and licorice in a coffee grinder—you don't need a fine powder. Store in a jar.

Make tea using 1 tsp. per mug infused for 5–10 minutes (p.15). Take 1–3 times daily to improve circulation.

Kidney-Strengthening Tea

A daily drink to support the kidneys.

INGREDIENTS
- ¾ oz. dried corn silk
- ¾ oz. dried nettle leaves

MAKES & KEEPS
Makes 1½-oz. herb mixture.
Keeps up to 1 year.

METHOD
Mix the herbs together. Make tea using 1 tbsp. to a teapot of boiling water.

Drink over the day.

Corn silk is the dried stamens seen on ears of corn—if you pick fresh or buy with the outer leaves still on, you see these long, thin pale yellow/green strands all around the cob. Remove them and lay to dry on a flat tray in a warm, dark place. When dry, they look like brown hair. Break them up and mix with the nettles.

Chilblain Oil

Courtesy of Sue Wine

INGREDIENTS
- 1 tbsp. vegetable oil (any, but almond and sesame work well)

Essential oils:
- 5 drops geranium
- 1 drop lavender
- 1 drop rosemary

MAKES & KEEPS
Makes 1 tbsp. for 1 application.
Use immediately.

METHOD
Mix the oils together and rub into chilblains when they are sore.

Equinox Tea for the Changing Seasons

Courtesy of Christine Herren-Valette

This tea helps to prepare for the important transition from winter to spring, and summer to fall—key times when people fall ill, as the body tries to go through a powerful detoxification process.

INGREDIENTS
Dried herbs:

- ¼ cup nettle tops
- 3 tbsp. downy birch leaves
- 2 tbsp. marigold flowers
- 1 tbsp. blackcurrant leaves
- 1 tbsp. meadowsweet flowers

MAKES & KEEPS
Makes 1 oz. herb mixture.
Keeps up to 1 year.

METHOD
Mix the herbs together and make a tea using 1 tsp. per mug of boiling water (p.15).

Take 2–3 times daily.

Honey, Lemon & Ginger for Colds

Courtesy of Sue Wine

INGREDIENTS
- 1-inch piece fresh ginger root
- 2 tsp. honey
- juice of ½ lemon

MAKES & KEEPS
1 mug.
Drink immediately.

METHOD
Peel and slice the ginger thinly. Place in a mug of boiling water, then add the other ingredients. Let brew for 5–10 minutes, then drink (you can also eat the pieces of ginger). It will make you sweat and banish your head cold.

63

Hyssop Cough Syrup

Courtesy of Teri Evans

INGREDIENTS
- ¾ cup + 2 tbsp. honey
- ¼ cup hot water
- 2 tbsp. dried hyssop, moistened with 1 tbsp. hot water
- 1 tsp. anise seeds, crushed

MAKES & KEEPS
Makes about 8½ fl. oz.
Keeps up to 1 year in the refrigerator until opened.

METHOD
Heat the honey and water gently in a saucepan until syrupy. Then let simmer for 5 minutes, regularly skimming off any scum that forms.

Next, add the hyssop and anise seeds. Stir, cover, and simmer for 30 minutes. Remove the lid and let cool slightly before straining into a jar.

Adults: Take 1 tbsp. up to 6 times daily.

Children: Take 1 tbsp. up to 4 times daily.

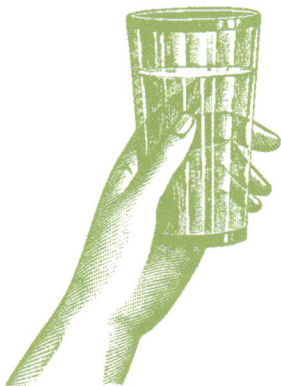

Turmeric Honey Antibiotic

To help your body fight any infection

INGREDIENTS
- 1 jar of honey
- 1 jar the same size of ground turmeric

KEEPS
2 years.

METHOD
Empty both jars into a bowl and mix thoroughly. Return the mixture to the original jars. Handle turmeric carefully, because it can stain.

Adults: Take 1 tsp. 3–4 times daily.

Children: Take ½ tsp. 3 times daily.

Birch Aromatic Syrup for Coughs & Sore Throats

Courtesy of Johanna Herzog

INGREDIENTS
- 2 cups vodka
- 2 handfuls of fresh birch leaves or leaves and buds
- 2 cups sugar (white or brown)

MAKES & KEEPS
Makes about 26 fl. oz.
Keeps indefinitely.

METHOD
Mix all the ingredients together in a saucepan and let them simmer gently for about 5 minutes. Strain and bottle while the syrup is still hot.

Adults: Take 1–2 tsp. every 4 hours.

Thyme & Licorice Cough Syrup

Courtesy of Joe Nasr

INGREDIENTS

- 2 oz. dried licorice root, chopped
- 6 cups hot water
- ¾ oz. dried rubbed thyme leaf
- white or brown sugar, variable amount
- 2 tbsp. + 1 tsp. pure vegetable glycerin

MAKES & KEEPS

Makes about 34 fl. oz.
Keeps at least 1 year.

METHOD

In a saucepan, soak the licorice root in the hot water for 1 hour. Cover with a lid, switch on the heat, and simmer for 25 minutes.

Turn off the heat. Mix in the thyme leaf and let cool.

Strain the liquid through cheesecloth and measure the liquid's exact weight. Stir an equal amount of the sugar thoroughly into the liquid.

Heat the mixture gently to around body temperature—lukewarm—and stir at this heat until the sugar is dissolved. Then mix in the glycerin and remove from the heat. Pour into bottles and seal when cooled.

Adults: Take 1–3 tsp. 2–3 times daily after meals

Children: Take ½–1 tsp. 2–3 times daily after meals.

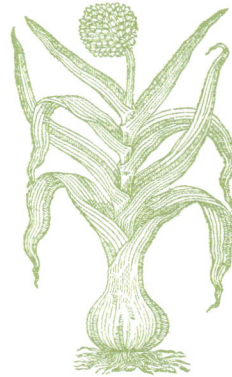

Garlic & Echinacea Infection-Busting Tincture

Growing your own echinacea if you can is a good idea, because it is particularly effective as a fresh tincture but is expensive to buy.

INGREDIENTS

- 1 oz. dried echinacea root, or ⅔ cup fresh roots and tops, chopped
- 2 heads garlic, peeled and crushed
- 2 cups vodka

MAKES & KEEPS

Makes almost 2 cups.
Keeps 2 years.

METHOD

Put all the ingredients into a large, lidded jar. Make a tincture (pp.18–19).

Adults: Take 1 tsp. 3–5 times daily for acute infections.

Children (under 12): Take 10–20 drops in a little cooled boiled water.

Antiviral Elder

Courtesy of ChaNan Bonser

An alcohol-free tincture. Use to prevent any viral infection or to aid recovery.

INGREDIENTS
- 6–8 heads fresh elderflowers
- 2 cups pure vegetable glycerin
- juice of 2 lemons
- 6–8 heads fresh elderberries

MAKES & KEEPS
Makes about 2 cups.
Keeps 1 year.

METHOD
Pick the elderflowers off the heads and put straight into a bowl. Cover the flowers with the glycerin, making sure they are completely covered. Add the lemon juice.

Put into a jar. Let sit for at least 1 month, shaking at least once a day, while you wait for the elderberries to ripen. When the elderberries are ripe, remove the berries from the stems and place the berries into a jar. Separately, strain the elderflower mixture through a strainer and pour the liquid over the elderberries, making sure they are all covered. Stir well and mash the mixture. Let sit for at least an additional 1 month, shaking every day.

After this time, strain the liquid again through cheesecloth, and rebottle.

Take 1 tsp. as required, either as it is or diluted in your favorite drink.

— Tip —

PICK YOUR ELDERFLOWERS ON
A DRY DAY, IDEALLY AFTER ANY DEW
HAS BEEN BURNED OFF.

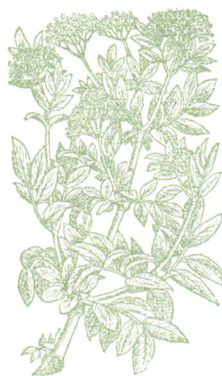

Barrier Bar for Busy Hands

Courtesy of Annie Powell

Protects hardworking hands from dry skin.

INGREDIENTS
- ⅔ cup virgin olive oil
- ⅔ cup grated beeswax
- 25 drops lavender or chamomile essential oil (or a mix of the two)

YOU WILL NEED:
- SHALLOW MUFFIN PANS
- WAX PAPER AND BROWN PAPER

MAKES & KEEPS
Makes 4–6 bars.
Keeps at least 1 year.

METHOD
In a double boiler or water bath, gently melt the olive oil and beeswax over low heat. Mix together thoroughly.

Remove from heat and add the essential oil(s). Pour into muffin pans and let cool. Turn out and wrap in wax paper, then brown paper.

Elderberry Oxymel

This remedy is an excellent vitamin C tonic and antiviral. Good for all ages, except for babies under one year of age because it contains honey, it can also help arthritis and rheumatic problems. It tastes wonderful with hot water and also makes a refreshing drink when made with sparkling water.

INGREDIENTS
- 7–8 heads fresh elderberries
- 3 cups Apple Cider Vinegar (p.165)
- 2½ cups unpasteurized honey

MAKES & KEEPS
Makes about 1 quart.
Keeps 1–2 years until opened, then keep in the refrigerator and use within 6 months.

METHOD
Gather the elderberries when they are ripe. Use to make an infused vinegar (p.19).

Pour the liquid into a saucepan and heat gently. Add the honey and stir it until it dissolves, taking the pan off the heat after 2 minutes. Do not boil, because this would destroy some of the honey's powerful properties. Pour into bottles.

Take 1 tsp. daily to prevent colds and flu. To treat them, take 1 tsp. 3–4 times daily.

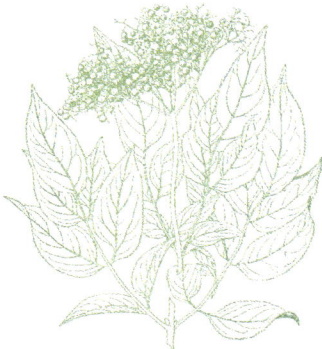

Elders' Sherry Tonic

This tonic is a tincture to help older bodies stay healthy and strong. There is a variation for women and men, using different types of ginseng.

INGREDIENTS
- 1 oz. dried milk vetch root
- ¾ oz. dried nettle tops
- 1 oz. dried ginkgo
- ½ cup unsulfured (brown) dried apricots, chopped
- 3 cups of your favorite sherry
- for men: 1 oz. dried ginseng root or American ginseng
- for women: 1 oz. dried Siberian ginseng root
- 6 tbsp. + 2 tsp./100ml hawthorn tincture (store-bought or Mother of the Heart Tincture, p.75)
- ¾ cup + 5 tsp. elderberry syrup or Antiviral Elder (opposite)

MAKES & KEEPS
Makes about 1 quart.
Keeps 2 years.

METHOD
Grind the roots to a coarse powder in a coffee grinder and place in a jar. Add the nettles, ginkgo, ginseng, and apricots, and cover with the sherry.

Let sit in a cool, dark place for 3 weeks, turning daily. Strain well and add the hawthorn tincture and elderberry syrup before bottling.

Take 1–2 tbsp. in a little water daily.

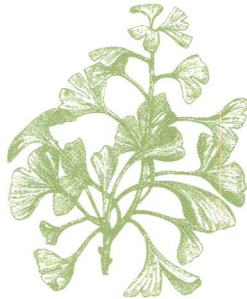

Elders' Alcohol-Free Tonic

INGREDIENTS
- 1 quart water
- 1 oz. dried milk vetch root
- ¾ oz. dried nettle leaf
- 1 oz. dried gingko
- for men: 1 oz. dried ginseng root or American ginseng
- for women: 1 oz. dried Siberian ginseng root
- ½ cup unsulfured (brown) dried apricots, chopped
- 1 (12-oz.) jar of honey
- ¾ cup Hawthorn Flower Syrup (p.157)
- ¾ cup elderberry syrup (p.20) or Antiviral Elder (p.66)

MAKES & KEEPS
Makes 1 quart.
Keeps 1 year until opened, then in the refrigerator for 1 month.

METHOD
Decoct the herbs and apricots in the water, boiling for 10 minutes (p.15). Let cool, strain, and press, then simmer the liquid for 10–15 minutes to reduce it to 2½ cups. Add the honey and continue to gently heat for 2–3 minutes, stirring to dissolve the honey, then mix in the Hawthorn Flower Syrup and add the elderberry syrup or Antiviral Elder. Bottle into 5 or more small bottles.

Take 1–2 tbs daily in water.

Brain Booster

There is some evidence that these ingredients are beneficial to the brain and could help prevent dementia.

INGREDIENTS
- 1 (12-oz.) jar of extra virgin coconut oil
- 1 oz. dried ground rosemary
- 2 oz. dried ground gingko

MAKES & KEEPS
Makes 15 oz.
Keeps up to 1 year.

METHOD
Stand the jar of coconut oil in a bowl of warm water to melt it.

Mix the rosemary and gingko together in a bowl, then pour the melted coconut oil over the mixture. Stir well and pour into jars.

Take 2–3 tsp. twice daily for maximum effect.

Coconut Inflammation Beater

Ginger and turmeric have been shown to have powerful anti-inflammatory properties, helping to prevent and cure many degenerative diseases. Coconut oil also has healing properties, reducing inflammation, improving metabolism, and nourishing the brain. It is a pleasant and easy way to take in the spices.

INGREDIENTS
- 1 (12-oz.) jar of extra virgin coconut oil
- 4 oz. ground turmeric
- 2 oz. ground ginger

MAKES & KEEPS
Makes 18 oz.
Keeps up to 1 year.

METHOD
Melt the coconut oil in a double boiler or bain-marie. Mix the turmeric and ginger in well and pour into jars.

Take 2 tsp. twice daily.

Bedsore & Blister Preventive

Rub this rubbing alcohol tincture into the skin to toughen it and to help prevent bedsores and blisters.

INGREDIENTS
- 10–15 fresh marigold flowers
- 1 small bunch of fresh sage leaves
- 1 small bunch of fresh lavender, stripped from stems
- 1 small bunch of fresh thyme, stripped from stems
- 1 quart rubbing alcohol

MAKES & KEEPS
Makes 1 quart.
Keeps indefinitely.

METHOD
Make a tincture from the herbs and rubbing alcohol (pp.18–19).

Rub into any areas of skin that need toughening, 2–3 times daily.

— *Tip* —

THE ACT OF GENTLY RUBBING
THE SKIN IMPROVES CIRCULATION
AND SO HELPS PREVENT BEDSORES.
FOR DELICATE SKIN, APPLY A HEALING
OINTMENT OR CREAM FREQUENTLY.

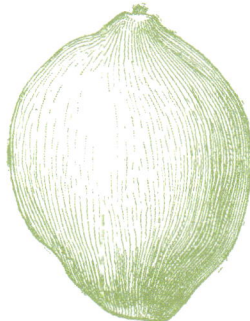

WELL-BEING TEAS

A great way of enhancing your well-being is to get into the habit of drinking herbal teas daily.

The following recipes are for dried herb mixtures that can be made into teas.

All dried herb mixtures should be stored in airtight jars away from the light—they'll keep at their best for up to a year this way.

To make the tea, mix 1–2 tsp. of the dried herb mixture into a mug of boiling water and leave to infuse (p.15). Once teas are made, they should be consumed immediately for best results.

Sleepy Tea

This tea will calm a wide-awake mind.

INGREDIENTS
- ¾ oz. passionflower
- 2 oz. valerian
- ¾ oz. lemon balm
- ½ oz. lavender

MAKES
Makes 4-oz. herb mixture.

METHOD
Drink a mug of sleepy tea half an hour before bed every night.

Antistress Tea

INGREDIENTS
- ¾ oz. lemon balm
- ¾ oz. wood betony
- ¾ oz. oatstraw
- ¾ oz. skullcap
- ¾ oz. vervain
- ¼ oz. lavender

MAKES
Makes 4-oz. herb mixture.

METHOD
Drink 1–3 mugs daily, with honey to sweeten, if required.

Cheering Tea

Courtesy of Dedj Leibbrandt
This colorful tea will bring a smile to your face.

INGREDIENTS
- ½ oz. lavender flowers
- ¼ oz. cornflowers
- ¼ oz. marigold petals
- ½ oz. lime flowers
- ½ oz. sage
- 2 tsp. dill seeds
- 1 tsp. poppy seeds

MAKES
Makes 2¼-oz. herb mixture.

METHOD
Drink 2–4 mugs daily.

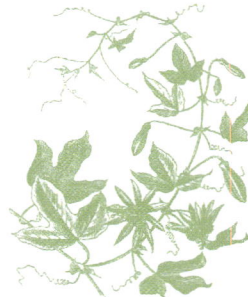

Grief Tea

The cure for grief is to mourn—to let feelings surface, acknowledge them, let tears flow, and wash away the grief. This is a tea to help that process happen in a gentle way.

INGREDIENTS
- ½ oz. **lemon balm**
- ½ oz. **rosebuds or petals**
- ½ oz. **heather flowering tops**

MAKES
Makes 1½-oz. herb mixture.

METHOD
Drink 3–5 mugs daily.

Pregnancy Tea

Take this tea during the last 3 months of pregnancy to strengthen and tone the womb, and your mind and heart, in preparation for birth.

INGREDIENTS
- 2 oz. **raspberry leaves**
- 2 oz. **rosebuds**

MAKES
Makes 4-oz. herb mixture.

METHOD
Drink 1–2 mugs daily.

In the last 3 weeks of pregnancy, add 2 oz. lady's mantle to the mix.

Continue to take the tea daily for at least 1 month after the baby is born to help the womb return to its normal size and recover its tone.

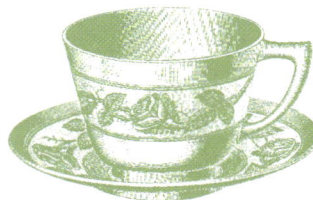

Quick Wake Up

Get going without caffeine!

INGREDIENTS
- 1 mug of rosemary tea (made by infusing 1 tsp. dried rosemary in 1 mug of boiling water for 10 minutes, then straining)
- ½ tsp. **cayenne pepper**

MAKES
Makes 1 mug. Drink immediately.

METHOD
Stir the cayenne pepper into the warm rosemary tea and drink. You're off!

Oak Bud Remedy for Strength

If you have never tried "tree hugging," start now. Lean right into the oak to connect with its deep strength and power of endurance, as you ask the tree to lend you its strength.

INGREDIENTS
- about 100 **oak buds**
- 1 cup **brandy**

MAKES & KEEPS
Makes 1 cup. Keeps for 2 years.

METHOD
Make a tincture with the oak buds and brandy (pp.18–19).

Decant the strained tincture into a small dropper bottle and take 1 drop any time extra courage and strength is needed.

MASSAGE OILS

Massage is a particularly powerful tool for keeping well. "Rubbing" was considered a vital part of a physician's work in Europe before the Dark Ages, when much useful medical knowledge was lost, and it is still integral to Chinese medicine and Ayurveda. The following recipes blend various oils for healing massage. They can be used as oils, or made into a soft balm with a little beeswax for a no-spill version.

Oils or balms should be stored in airtight containers away from the light, and will keep for up to a few months, depending on how long the base oil keeps (see infused oils, page 20).

To use, put a little of the oil or balm into your hands and massage into skin.

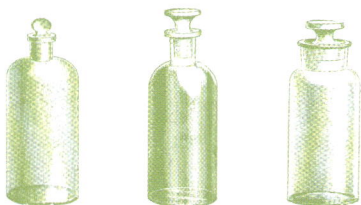

Stimulating Massage Oil

This is good for warming and stimulating muscles, joints, and skin.

INGREDIENTS
- ⅓ cup almond oil infused with rosemary leaves, dried or fresh (p.20)
- 2 tbsp. mustard seed oil

Essential oils:
- 5 drops rosemary
- 5 drops black pepper
- 5 drops cardamom
- 5 drops ginger

MAKES & KEEPS
Makes ⅓ cup.
Keeps 1–2 months.

METHOD
Mix the ingredients in a bottle and gently shake.

Relaxing Massage Oil

INGREDIENTS
- ½ cup Lavender-Infused Oil (opposite)

Essential oils:
- 10 drops lavender
- 10 drops clary sage

MAKES & KEEPS
Makes ½ cup.
Keeps 1–2 months.

METHOD
Mix the ingredients in a bottle and gently shake.

— Variation —

FOR A SENSUAL MASSAGE BALM,
USE ½ CUP OF ROSE AND JASMINE
INFUSED OIL (P.20) AND 10 DROPS EACH
OF JASMINE, SANDALWOOD, ROSE, AND
YLANG YLANG ESSENTIAL OILS.

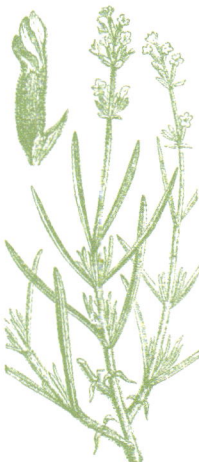

Stress-Busting Massage Balm

INGREDIENTS
- ½ cup Lavender-Infused Oil (right)
- 1½ tsp. grated beeswax

Essential oils:
- 10 drops lavender
- 10 drops sandalwood
- 10 drops cedarwood
- 10 drops bergamot

MAKES & KEEPS
Makes ½ cup.
Keeps around 3 months.

METHOD
Melt the beeswax into the infused oil in a double boiler or water bath. Add the essential oils and pour into a container.

Lavender-Infused Oil

Lavender is a relaxing and soothing herb with anti–inflammatory properties.

INGREDIENTS
- 1 oz. dried lavender flowers
- ¾ cup olive oil
- ¾ cup grapeseed oil

MAKES & KEEPS
Makes about 1½ cups.
Keeps around 6 months.

METHOD
Fill a jar with the best, most fragrant lavender flowers you can find. Cover with the olive and grapeseed oils. Let infuse for 3–4 weeks. Strain well and bottle.

Birch Massage Oil

Courtesy of Johanna Herzog

Soothing, for inflamed skin and cellulitis.

INGREDIENTS

- 3 cups oil or a mixture of oils of your choice (apricot kernel, macadamia, jojoba, pure almond oil, or coconut are some of my favorites)
- 2 handfuls of fresh birch leaves, chopped
- 3 tbsp. vodka
- grated zest of 1 lemon

MAKES & KEEPS

Makes about 3 cups.
Keeps 6–12 months.

METHOD

Put the ingredients into a jar. Let sit in a warm place for 3 weeks, then strain through cheesecloth and bottle the liquid. Shake well before use.

Fiery Muscle Rub

A deep heat rub for aches and pains.

INGREDIENTS

- 1 cup Fire Cider (p.165)
- 1 cup Hot Oil (p.155)

MAKES & KEEPS

Makes 2 cups. Keeps at least 12 months.

METHOD

Mix the ingredients together in a bottle. Shake before each use.

Caution

Wash your hands well after applying the Fiery Muscle Rub, because getting it in your eyes or anywhere delicate would really sting.

Stretch Mark Prevention Oil for Pregnant Women

Massage this oil into the abdomen and breasts before bedtime every day from the start of the second trimester. For the third trimester, also apply it in the morning.

INGREDIENTS

- 2 tbsp. Heal-All Marigold Oil (p.81)
- 2 tbsp. Comfrey Oil (p.80)
- 5 tsp. rosehip oil
- 2 tsp. evening primrose oil
- 1 tsp. vitamin E oil (or another 1 tsp. evening primrose oil)

Essential oils:
- 10 drops mandarin
- 10 drops lavender

MAKES & KEEPS

Makes just under ½ cup.
Keeps 6 months.

METHOD

Blend the oils in a bottle and use as much as required, as instructed above.

Mother of the Heart Tincture

Hawthorn, known in herbal medicine as "the mother of the heart," is used to support the heart and circulation for pretty much any condition. This is a simple tincture, with the added advantage of tasting good.

INGREDIENTS
- **2 large handfuls of fresh hawthorn berries (dried if you can't find fresh)**
- **3–4 cups vodka**

MAKES & KEEPS
Makes 3–3¾ cups.
Keeps at least 2 years.

METHOD
Make a tincture with the berries and vodka (pp.18–19).

Take 1 tsp. in water daily to help protect against heart disease.

Always consult a qualified health professional for advice if you have a heart condition.

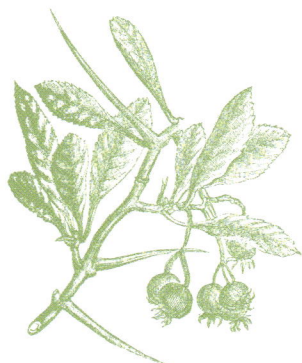

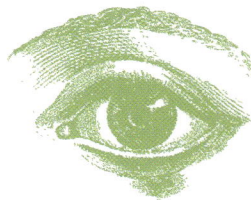

Clear Vision Drops

Courtesy of Sensory Solutions

Although these drops can be used to treat and prevent eye problems, they also have an effect on the "energetic" vision—our ability to see solutions and directions in life.

INGREDIENTS
Tinctures (pp.18–19):
- **2 tbsp./30ml bilberry tincture**
- **2 tbsp./30ml heather tincture**

MAKES & KEEPS
Makes ¼ cup.
Keeps 2 years.

METHOD
Mix the tinctures in a dropper bottle ready to take.

Take a few drops of the mixture 4 times daily. If you want, repeat an affirmation 3 times out loud as you do so. The affirmation should be related to what you want from the drops (for example, "I can see a clear path to the solution I seek"). It will thus connect you to their purpose every time you take them.

Agrimony Teachers' Gargle

Perfect for easing and restoring overworked throats.

INGREDIENTS
- 1 quart boiling water
- 1 oz. dried agrimony
- ½ oz. dried sage, chopped

MAKES & KEEPS
Makes about 4 cups.
Keeps 4 days in the refrigerator.

METHOD
Pour boiling water on the herbs and let sit until cold. Strain and press through a cheesecloth-lined funnel. Store the liquid in a bottle.

To use, dilute ½ mug with a little hot water. Gargle 3 times daily.

Marshmallow Cough Syrup

Courtesy of Teri Evans

INGREDIENTS
- 1 tbsp. chopped dried marshmallow root or leaves
- just under 2 cups water
- 1¾ cups brown sugar
- ¼ cup orange juice or juice of 1 lemon

MAKES & KEEPS
Makes about 17 fl. oz.
Keeps 1 year unopened; once opened, keeps 1–2 months in the refrigerator.

METHOD
Soak the marshmallow root or leaves in the water overnight. Strain in the morning, then simmer the liquid with the sugar for 5 minutes to make a thick syrup. Add the juice and bottle.

Take 1–2 tsp. as needed.

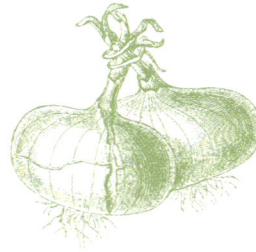

Quick Onion Cough Syrup

Courtesy of Lucy Wells

This syrup can help to soothe a cough and fight infection in the lungs.

INGREDIENTS
- 1–2 tbsp. brown sugar
- 1 onion

MAKES & KEEPS
Makes a small, variable amount—about 10 tsp. Use over 2–3 days.

METHOD
Put the sugar on a small plate or a saucer. Cut the onion and put onto the sugar, cut sides down.

Let sit for 24 hours. The sugar pulls out the onion's juices and together they make the syrup in the saucer.

Take 1 tsp. every 1–2 hours until the cough is soothed.

— Tip —
ACCORDING TO ONION LORE, A CUT ONION IN A ROOM WILL REMOVE ANY UNWANTED INFECTION/IMPURITY FROM THE AIR (THOUGH IT IS NOT RECOMMENDED FOR USE IN FOOD PREPARATIONS). PUTTING CUT ONION IN A SOCK AND HOLDING IT TO THE EAR CAN HELP GREATLY WITH EARACHE.

Ear Oil

Courtesy of Monika Ghent

Use this oil for earaches or to soften up ear wax so that it can be gently removed.

INGREDIENTS
- 2 tsp. coconut oil
- 2 tsp. jojoba oil

Infused oils (p.20):
- 2 tsp. marigold
- 2 tsp. St. John's wort
- 2 tsp. mullein flower

- oil from 3 (400 IU) vitamin E oil capsules

MAKES & KEEPS
Makes about ¼ cup.
Keeps 3–6 months.

METHOD
Gently melt the coconut oil, then mix with all the ingredients into a dropper bottle.

Shake the mixture well before using. Put 1–2 drops into each ear and close off the ear with a cotton ball. Keep in place overnight, removing the cotton ball the next morning.

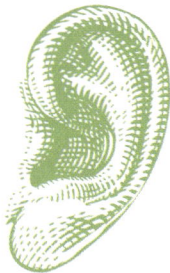

Mullein Pile Ointment

An old effective gardener's treatment for piles, or hemorrhoids, was bruising a fresh mullein leaf and putting it in your underwear. Mullein leaves are velvety soft, so it is probably nice; on the other hand, you may prefer this recipe.

INGREDIENTS
- ¾ oz. dried mullein leaves, or several fresh leaves, shredded
- 2 cups olive oil
- ¼ cup grated beeswax

MAKES & KEEPS
Makes about 2 cups.
Keeps up to 1 year.

METHOD
Make an infused oil by gently heating the mullein in the olive oil (p.20).

Gently heat the beeswax and the infused oil together in a double boiler or water bath until the wax has melted, then pour into jars. Place the lids on loosely and tighten when the mixture has cooled.

To use, wash carefully after each bowel movement and apply ointment. Can be applied 3–4 times daily in addition.

— *Tip* —

ANY INFUSED OIL CAN BE MADE INTO AN OINTMENT USING THE METHOD ABOVE.

FIRST-AID PLANT POWER

Nature's kingdom is abundant in all kinds of powerful remedies for injuries, emergencies, and life's ups and downs. This chapter is packed with home remedies for soothing and healing cuts, bruises, breaks, and strains, and for treating everyday ailments, such as colds and flu, headaches, hay fever, and stomach upsets.

Antiseptic Mist

Courtesy of Louise Idoux

INGREDIENTS

- 2 tbsp. + 2 tsp. lavender aromatic water (p.15)
- 2 tbsp. + 2 tsp. bay aromatic water (p.15)
- 2 tsp./10ml myrrh tincture (see box below and pp.18–19)
- 2 tsp./10ml calendula tincture (pp.18–19)
- ½ tsp. raw honey (preferably manuka)
- 1 drop tea tree essential oil

MAKES & KEEPS

Makes just under ½ cup.
Keeps up to 18 months.

METHOD

Mix together in a spray bottle or mister.

Spray once or twice directly on to wounds, twice daily.

— Tip —

YOU CAN MAKE YOUR OWN TINCTURES BY FOLLOWING THE GUIDELINES ON PP.18–19. YOU CAN USE VODKA TO MAKE ALL TINCTURES, EXCEPT FOR TINCTURE OF MYRRH, WHICH IS MADE FROM MYRRH RESIN AND REQUIRES 90 PERCENT ALCOHOL—YOU CAN GET EVERCLEAR GRAIN ALCOHOL THAT IS 190 PROOF FOR THIS PURPOSE.

Honey & Marigold Graze Remedy

Try this instead of painfully picking gravel out of a graze. Honey is antiseptic, with strong healing properties; combined with the amazing marigold, it makes for miraculous healing.

INGREDIENTS

- 20 or so fresh marigold flowers (or ⅓ oz. dried)
- 1 (12-oz.) jar of honey

MAKES & KEEPS

Makes 12 oz.
Keeps 1–2 years or more.

METHOD

Put the marigold flowers into a jar. Pour the honey over them, up to the top. Let sit for 2–3 weeks, or until you need it (there is no need to take the flowers out of the honey).

To use, slather the honey all over the grazed area. Cover with a large bandage and leave overnight. The next day, carefully peel off the bandage. The honey will have pulled out all the tiny stones, leaving the wound clean.

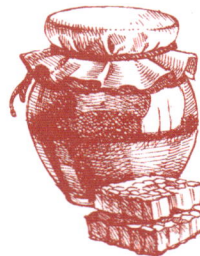

Quick Chamomile Eye Poultice for Sore Eyes

INGREDIENTS
- 1–2 chamomile tea bags
- 2 tbsp. boiling water

MAKES & KEEPS
This makes enough for one or both eyes. For immediate use.

METHOD
Put the tea bags into a small bowl and cover with the boiling water. When cooled to just warm, lightly drain the bags.

Lie down and place the bags over closed eyes for 5–15 minutes.

Antibacterial Honey

This do-it-yourself antibiotic is powerful. It can be taken for any infection, especially one of the ears, nose, throat, lungs, and teeth.

INGREDIENTS
- 2 heads garlic, peeled and crushed
- 1 cup fresh thyme leaves and flowers, removed from stems (or rubbed, if using dried)
- up to 1 (12-oz.) jar of honey

MAKES & KEEPS
Makes 12 oz.
Keeps at least 3–6 months.

METHOD
Mix the garlic and thyme in an empty 12-oz. jar. Pour the honey over the mixture, making sure all is covered.

Adults: Take 1 tsp. 3–4 times daily.

Children: Take ½ tsp. 3 times daily.

Ulcer-Healing Honey

INGREDIENTS
Dried ground herbs:
- 1 oz. licorice root
- 1 oz. myrrh resin
- 1 oz. marigold flowers
- ¼ cup raw honey (preferably manuka)

MAKES & KEEPS
Makes 1¼ cups.
Keeps for years.

METHOD
Mix all the ingredients thoroughly and store in a jar. Apply frequently to canker sores and other open sores that are not healing well.

Take 1 tsp. 2–3 times daily for ulcers in the digestive system.

Spray for Strained or Sore Throats

INGREDIENTS
- 2 drops thyme essential oil
- ½ tsp. pure vegetable glycerin
- 2 tsp./10ml sage tincture (pp.18–19)
- 2 tsp./10ml echinacea tincture (pp.18–19)
- 1 tbsp. elderberry, rowan, or rose hip syrup, or a mixture (p.21)
- 4 tsp. boiled water

MAKES & KEEPS
Makes 2 (1-fl.-oz.) spray bottles.
Keeps 3–6 months.

METHOD
Beat the thyme essential oil into the glycerin. Slowly add the sage tincture, echinacea tincture, syrup, and the boiled water, beating as you pour. Mix well, then bottle in small spray bottles for ease of use.

To use, spray directly into the back of the mouth as often as required.

Simple Turnip Cough Syrup

Courtesy of Anne Chiotis

An expectorant to help your lungs clear themselves of mucus.

INGREDIENTS
- 1 fresh turnip
- plenty of brown sugar

MAKES & KEEPS
Makes a variable amount.
Best used fresh, but keeps up to 2–3 weeks in the refrigerator.

METHOD
Hollow out the center of a turnip, leaving 1¼–1½ inches of flesh around the edge. Fill it with brown sugar and let sit for 12 hours. A delectable syrup will form as the sugar draws the juice out of the turnip. You can simply store the turnip in the refrigerator, using it as your "cup," or decant the syrup into a jar.

Take 1–3 tsp. 3 times daily.

Comfrey Oil

This makes a powerful healing oil. Dried comfrey leaves work best; fresh ones are juicy and hold too much water to use in an oil.

INGREDIENTS
- 2 oz. dried comfrey leaves
- 2 cups olive oil or other vegetable oil

MAKES & KEEPS
Makes just under 2 cups.
Keeps 3–12 months.

METHOD
Make as described for the Heal-All Marigold Oil (opposite).

Use in creams, ointments, and liniments for healing connective tissue.

Intensive Skin Repair Balm

Courtesy of Iain Stewart

This solid, waxy balm for cracked skin, especially on hands and heels, is popular with climbers.

INGREDIENTS
- 8 tsp. grated beeswax
- 2 tbsp. jojoba oil
- 7 tbsp. grapeseed oil
- 1 tbsp. Comfrey Oil (left)

Essential oils:
- 24 drops tangerine
- 12 drops petitgrain
- 6 drops patchouli
- 6 drops black pepper
- 6 drops cypress
- 6 drops benzoin

- oil from 3 (400 IU) vitamin E capsules

YOU WILL NEED
· 6 (1-oz.) SILICONE MOLDS

MAKES & KEEPS
Makes 6 blocks of 1-oz. blocks.
Keeps for years.

METHOD
Place the beeswax, jojoba, grapeseed, and Comfrey Oil in a double boiler or water bath. Heat for a couple of minutes, until the wax has melted.

Let cool for 5 minutes, stirring from time to time. Then add the essential oils and vitamin E, mixing well.

Put the mixture into silicone molds and let sit overnight. It will set hard. Remove from the molds and store.

Heal-All Marigold Oil

Pot marigold, often known by its Latin name
Calendula officialis, *has many excellent healing
qualities and is wonderfully easy to grow. Its infused
oil is used alone or in many healing and nourishing
balms, ointments, and creams. This recipe uses the hot
method, double infused.*

INGREDIENTS
- **4 cups pot marigold flowers, freshly picked
(or 1 oz. dried)**
- **just under 2 cups olive oil or other
vegetable oil**

MAKES & KEEPS
Makes about 1⅔ cups.
Keeps 3–12 months.

METHOD
Put half the marigolds into a double boiler.
Heat gently in the oil. Keep on especially low
heat, just warming the oil really, for 3 hours.

Remove from heat and let cool. When cool,
strain and press through a strainer or funnel
lined with cheesecloth. Compost the remainder
of the herbs.

Add the remaining marigolds to the infused oil.
Repeat the simmering process for another
2 hours, then let cool and strain again. This
is now a double-infused oil (p.20).

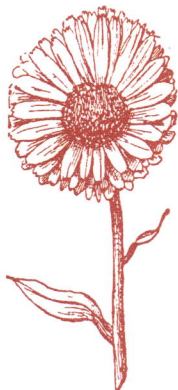

Heal-All Marigold Cream

*Use this cream made from pot marigolds for its
antibacterial and soothing effects.*

INGREDIENTS
Oil fraction:
- **6 tbsp. + 2 tsp. Heal-All Marigold Oil
(left)**
- **½ cup emulsifying wax**

Water fraction:
- **¾ cup + 5 tsp. strong marigold tea (p.15)**
- **6 tbsp. + 2 tsp./100ml marigold tincture
(pp.18–19)**

Extras:
- **½ tsp. benzoin tincture/2ml (Friar's
Balsam)**

MAKES & KEEPS
Makes just under 2 cups.
Keeps 6–12 months in the refrigerator.

METHOD
Make the cream following the method for
Comfrey Cream for Speedy Healing (p.82).

— Variation —

FOR A MULTIPURPOSE
ANTISEPTIC CREAM, STIR IN
½ TSP. LAVENDER ESSENTIAL
OIL RIGHT AT THE END OF
THE PROCESS.

Comfrey Cream for Speedy Healing

Courtesy of Dedj Leibbrandt

Read the cream-making instructions (pp. 20–21) before you start. Creams made using emulsifying wax are usually foolproof.

INGREDIENTS
Oil fraction:
- 6 tbsp. + 2 tsp. Comfrey Oil (p.80)
- ½ cup emulsifying wax

Water fraction:
- ¾ cup + 5 tsp. strong comfrey tea (p.15)
- 6 tbsp. + 2 tsp./100ml comfrey tincture (pp.18–19)

Extras:
- ½ tsp./2ml benzoin tincture (Friar's Balsam)

MAKES & KEEPS
Makes just under 2 cups.
Keeps 6–12 months in the refrigerator.

METHOD
Gently heat the oil fraction in a double boiler or water bath. Once the wax has melted, add the tea. Keep the mixture on the heat if it needs to remelt.

Next, add the water fraction and then put the pan in a basin of cold water to quickly cool it—his is called a cold water bath. Whisk the mixture constantly until it emulsifies, which takes 3–4 minutes with a handheld mixer. Then mix in the benzoin tincture (to preserve the cream) and pour into jars.

Apply liberally to any injury where the skin remains unbroken.

— Variation —

THE COMFREY CREAM RECIPE CAN BE ADAPTED TO MAKE ANY CREAM, SUBSTITUTING DIFFERENT HERBS TO SUIT DIFFERENT PURPOSES. YOU CAN ALSO ADD ESSENTIAL OILS FOR THEIR HEALING QUALITIES (UP TO ½ TSP. EACH) WHEN YOU ADD THE BENZOIN. SEE THE "HEAL-ALL MARIGOLD CREAM" FOR EXAMPLE (P.81), AND THE "STOP ITCH CREAM" (BELOW).

Stop Itch Cream

Courtesy of Dedj Leibbrandt

INGREDIENTS
Oil fraction:
- 3 tbsp. + 1 tsp. chickweed infused oil (made using ¼ cup olive oil infused with 2 tbsp. chickweed)
- ¼ cup emulsifying wax

Water fraction:
- 6 tbsp. + 2 tsp. strong chickweed infusion (p.15)
- 3 tbsp. + 1 tsp./50ml chickweed tincture (pp.18–19)
- 30 drops peppermint essential oil
- 20 drops benzoin tincture (Friar's Balsam)

MAKES & KEEPS
Makes 8 oz.
Keeps 1 year.

METHOD
Make in the same way as Comfrey Cream for Speedy Healing (left), stirring in the peppermint oil with the benzoin tincture.

Apply liberally to ease itching as often as needed. Do not use on broken skin.

St. John's Wort Oil

This beautiful red infused oil with anti-inflammatory, healing, and antiviral action uses the sun's power to capture the healing properties of St. John's wort. You have to make this oil from freshly picked flowers, and it requires sunlight to develop properly.

INGREDIENTS
- **any size jar full of freshly picked St. John's wort flowers**
- **olive oil, for covering**

MAKES & KEEPS
Keeps 6–12 months.

METHOD
Pour the olive oil over your freshly picked flowers, right up to the top of jar.

Add the lid and place the jar in a sunny spot, turning daily. It takes 2–8 weeks to be ready, depending on how much sun it receives. You know it is ready because the oil turns deep red.

Strain, press, and wring out through a cheesecloth-lined strainer or funnel into a dark bottle. Compost the spent flowers.

Add more flowers and continue for a double infusion if desired, as for Heal-All Marigold Oil (p.81).

This oil is great for applying to herpes and shingles, and added to any anti-inflammatory cream, ointment, liniment, or rub.

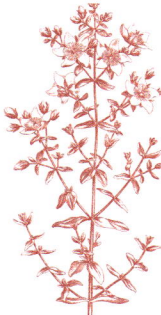

Antiseptic Healing Lotion

INGREDIENTS
Tinctures (pp.18–19):
- **¼ cup/60ml St. John's wort**
- **¼ cup/60ml marigold**

MAKES & KEEPS
Makes ½ cup.
Keeps 1–2 years.

METHOD
Mix the tinctures together.

Apply undiluted to bites and stings, cuts, grazes, acne, cold sores, and so on.

Dilute a few drops in a mug of water to wash infected skin 2–3 times daily.

Aloe Vera Instant Burn Remedy

Aloe vera is easy to grow. Its long leaves are full of a transparent gel that can be applied directly to burned skin, with immediate soothing and healing results.

INGREDIENTS
- **1 fresh aloe vera leaf**

MAKES & KEEPS
Makes enough for 1 application.
Use immediately.

METHOD
Cut the leaf lengthwise with a sharp knife.

Scrape out the gel and apply it straight to a burn.

— *Tip* —

LAVENDER ESSENTIAL OIL CAN ALSO BE APPLIED UNDILUTED TO EVEN SEVERE BURNS WITH EXCELLENT EFFECT.

Sage & Daisy Poultice for Bruises & Swellings

INGREDIENTS
- **fresh sage leaves**
- **fresh daisies**
- **vinegar to cover**

MAKES & KEEPS
Makes 1 application.
Use immediately.

METHOD
Gather enough herbs to cover the area. Gently heat the herbs and the vinegar together for about 5 mins. Do not boil.

Lay the herbs, still hot, out on a thin piece of cloth. Fold the cloth to a size big enough to cover the bruised area. Place it on the body, while the herbs are still hot but not in danger of burning. Wrap it with a towel to retain the heat.

Replace 1–2 times daily, as needed.

— Variation —

USE A VINEGAR INFUSED WITH SAGE, ROSEMARY, OR COMFREY (P.19) AS A VARIATION ON THE ABOVE.

Poultice for Broken Bones & Strains

Fresh comfrey root is a miraculous healer. Keep some in the freezer so that you have it on hand whenever you need it.

INGREDIENTS
- **fresh comfrey root**
- **about 3 tbsp. hot water**

YOU WILL NEED
- A BLENDER
- GAUZE AND MICROPORE TAPE

MAKES & KEEPS
Makes 1 application.
Fresh roots keep 2 weeks in the refrigerator.
Keeps 3–6 months in the freezer.

METHOD
Put enough comfrey root to cover the affected area in a blender, with the hot water to help it blend up. Mix to a smooth paste. If you don't have a blender, you can grate the roots.

Apply to the affected area. Cover the poultice with gauze and micropore tape to hold it in place.

It will become a hard, dry cast after a few days. At this point, remove the poultice, replacing it with a fresh application.

Do not use on open wounds.

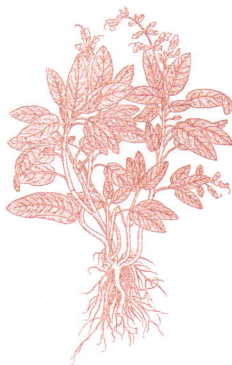

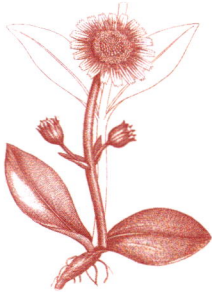

Ribwort Poultice for Infected Wounds

Courtesy of Eliot Cowan

A simple and highly effective cure.

INGREDIENTS
- **fresh ribwort plantain leaves**

MAKES & KEEPS
Makes 1 application.
Use immediately.

METHOD
Mash up the leaves (or chew them) to make a poultice.

Put the poultice on infected or suppurating wounds, and insect bites or stings. Change frequently.

— Tip —

YOU CAN USE DRIED LEAVES
FOR POULTICES—JUST ADD SOME
HOT WATER TO MAKE IT JUICY.

Canker Sore Cure

Courtesy of Eliot Cowan

An incredibly efficacious and fast-acting cure for canker sores in the mouth.

INGREDIENTS
- **small piece of golden thread root**

KEEPS
Use immediately.

METHOD
Place a small amount of the golden root between the gums or teeth and the sore. It is bitter, but keep sucking on it until the bitterness almost disappears, then remove.

Repeat until the sore is cured.

Daisy Bruise Ointment

You can use arnica instead of daisies.

INGREDIENTS
- **30–40 common daisy flowers**
- **⅓ cup olive oil**
- **1 tbsp. grated beeswax**

MAKES & KEEPS
Makes 4 oz..
Keeps 6–12 months.

METHOD
Make an infused oil with the daisies (p.20); you should end up with ½ cup of infused oil.

Gently heat the beeswax and the infused oil together until melted. Pour into jars.

Apply to bruises 3–6 times daily or as needed.

Jewelweed Salve for Skin Infections

Courtesy of Eliot Cowan

Jewelweed is not only a good remedy against fungal skin infections, such as athlete's foot, ringworm, pityriasis versicolor, and so on, but it is also an antidote to poison ivy when applied to the skin.

INGREDIENTS
- I handful of fresh jewelweed leaves, stems, and flowers
- I cup olive oil
- I oz. grated beeswax

MAKES & KEEPS
Makes I cup.
Keeps at least I year.

METHOD
Gently heat the jewelweed and olive oil to make an infused oil (p.20). The liquid will turn bright orange, the color of the flowers.

Strain the mixture. Then gently heat the beeswax into the oil to make a salve.

Apply the salve liberally and frequently to infected skin.

— Tip —
YOU CAN ALSO MAKE A TEA (P.15) FROM THE JEWELWEED AND DAB THE COOLED LIQUID ON THE INFECTED AREA FREQUENTLY.

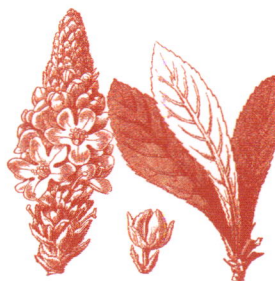

Mullein Flower Oil for Earache

You can make this oil using either the cold- or heat–infused method—see page 20.

INGREDIENTS
- just under I²⁄₃ cups mullein flowers, freshly picked
- just over ¾ cup olive oil

MAKES & KEEPS
Makes just over ¾ cup.
Keeps 3–6 months.

METHOD
Make an infused oil with the mullein flowers and olive oil (p.20). Once ready, store the bulk in a jar and a small amount in a dropper bottle for ease of administering the oil.

Put a few drops directly into the ear 3–6 times daily.

— Variation —
ADD ½–⅔ TSP. OF LAVENDER ESSENTIAL OIL, WHICH IS GOOD FOR TREATING AND PREVENTING INFECTIONS.

Cold & Flu Tea

This classic remedy helps to prevent a cold if you catch it early, as you begin to shiver and feel its onset. It stimulates the circulation and promotes sweating.

INGREDIENTS
Dried herbs:
- I oz. elderflowers
- I oz. peppermint leaves
- I oz. yarrow flowers

MAKES & KEEPS
Makes 3-oz. herb mixture.
Keeps I year.

METHOD
Mix the ingredients thoroughly. Make tea (p.15) using 2–3 tsp. per mug of boiling water, infused for 5 minutes.

Drink freely.

— Tip —

MAKE ICE POPS WITH THIS TEA: MAKE 2 CUPS COLD & FLU TEA AND SWEETEN WITH HONEY TO TASTE. LEAVE TO COOL, THEN FREEZE IN POPSICLE OR ICE-CUBE MOLDS. SUCK ON THEM TO CALM SORE THROATS AND FEVERS.

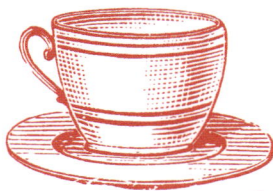

Basil Snifterchief

Courtesy of Sue Wine

A surprisingly effective remedy to protect against, and treat, sore throats and viral colds.

INGREDIENTS
- 5 drops basil essential oil

MAKES & KEEPS
Makes I application.
Use the same day.

METHOD
Drop the basil oil onto a handkerchief. Keep it in your pocket or under your pillow and sniff often. Just smell the oil—do not touch the handkerchief to your skin.

Xmas Survival Tummy Tonic

Helps to settle the stomach after overindulging in rich foods.

INGREDIENTS
Dried ground herbs:
- ½ oz. angelica root
- ½ oz. chamomile
- ½ oz. licorice
- ½ oz. marshmallow root
- ½ oz. artichoke roots or milk thistle seeds

- I (12-oz.) jar of honey (optional)

MAKES & KEEPS
Makes 14½ oz.
Keeps I year.

METHOD
Mix the ground herbs thoroughly with the honey to make a paste or thick syrup.

Take I–2 tsp. in a glass or cup of hot water I–3 times daily for as long as needed.

Headache Powders

A preventive for chronic, regular headache and migraines.

INGREDIENTS

Dried ground herbs:
- 1 oz. ginkgo
- ½ oz. feverfew leaves
- 1 oz. valerian root
- ½ oz. ginger root

MAKES & KEEPS

Makes 3-oz. herb mixture.
Keeps 1 year.

METHOD

Simply mix all the herbs together and store in a jar.

Take 1 tsp. in hot water 2–3 times daily as a headache preventive.

Caution

Dehydration is a common cause of headaches, and magnesium deficiency can be a factor in migraines. If you experience regular headaches or migraines, consult an herbalist for tailor-made treatment.

Herbal Aspirin

Aspirin was first found in willow bark. It has been used for centuries as a pain-killer for headaches and other pains, and to bring down fevers.

INGREDIENTS

Dried ground herbs:
- 2 oz. willow bark
- 1 oz. lavender
- 2 oz. valerian
- 1 oz. skullcap

MAKES & KEEPS

Makes 6-oz. herb mixture. Keeps 1 year.

METHOD

Mix the herbs together well.

Take 1–2 tsp. of the powder in a mug of water up to 4 times daily.

Homage to Hildegard Hangover Cure

Courtesy of Teri Evans

This hangover cure is based on a medieval recipe by Hildegard of Bingen. It draws upon herbs used at that time for "swimmings of the head" and so forth.

INGREDIENTS

Tinctures (pp.18–19):
- 5 tsp./25ml chamomile
- 4 tsp./20ml holy thistle
- 4 tsp./20ml milk thistle
- 1 tbsp./15ml meadowsweet
- 1 tbsp./15ml wood betony
- ½ tsp./2ml ginger

MAKES & KEEPS

Makes just under ½ cup. Keeps 2 years.

METHOD

Mix the tinctures together and store.

Take 1 tsp. twice before midday, dissolved in 2½ cups water.

Homemade Tiger Balm

Courtesy of Catherine Johnson

A famous pungent pain-killer, originally from Burma. Apply a small amount to the temples to ease headaches or rub on to itching insect bites or tired muscles.

INGREDIENTS
- just under ½ cup hemp oil
- 1 tbsp. grated or small pieces beeswax

Essential oils:
- 100 drops/1 tsp. peppermint
- 60 drops/½ tsp. camphor oil
- 80 drops/⅔ tsp. wintergreen
- 60 drops/ ½ tsp. lavender
- 60 drops/½ tsp. eucalyptus

MAKES & KEEPS
Makes ½ cup.
Keeps 6–12 months.

METHOD
Gently melt the hemp oil and beeswax in a double boiler or water bath. Let cool for 5 minutes, then add the essential oils.

Stir well and pour the balm into a jar.

Keep it away from eyes.

Hay Fever Mead

If you can, start taking herbal hay–fever medicine a week or two before you usually start to feel the allergy. Ideally, make the mead from fresh herbs, otherwise dried will do.

INGREDIENTS
- 1 handful of elderflowers
- 1 handful of thyme leaves and flowers
- 1 handful of eyebright, leaves and flowers
- 1 handful of plantain leaves
- 1 handful of chamomile flowers
- 1 handful of nettle tops
- 2½ cups mead

MAKES & KEEPS
Makes 2⅓ cups.
Keeps over 1 year.

METHOD
Gather the herbs, if using fresh.

Remove from stems, then cut up or shred.

Mix the herbs together and make a tincture using the mead (pp.18–19).

If already experiencing hay fever, take 1–2 tsp. 3 times daily. To prevent onset, try ½–1 tsp.

Children can take 10–20 drops 3 times daily.

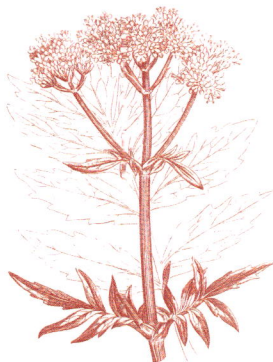

FIRST-AID KIT FOR TRAVELERS

For traveling, it is always good to take your own remedies with you, because you may not be able to easily source some herbs while you are away. Remember that if you are flying, there will be restrictions on taking liquids and pastes in your hand luggage.

Travel Sickness Candies

Read the candy-making section (pp. 21–22) before attempting this recipe.

INGREDIENTS
- 1 handful of fresh chopped ginger root
- 1⅔ cups water
- 1½ cups brown sugar
- 2 tbsp. butter or almond oil

MAKES & KEEPS
Makes 20–40 candies.
Keeps 3–4 weeks.

METHOD
Boil the ginger in the water for 20 minutes. Strain and measure. If necessary, reduce the liquid further by simmering with the lid off. You're aiming for just over ¾ cup.

With the liquid still over the heat, add the sugar and boil until you reach "hard-ball" stage (p.22). Remove from the heat and stir in the butter or oil.

High-Flier Candies for Anxious Fliers

Read the candy-making section (pp. 21–22) before attempting this recipe.

INGREDIENTS
Dried herbs:
- 1 oz. valerian root
- ½ oz. passionflower
- 1 oz. red clover (mildly blood thinning)

- 2 cups water
- 2 cups sugar

MAKES & KEEPS
Makes 40–70 candies.
Keeps 3–4 weeks in an airtight container.

METHOD
Boil the valerian, passionflower, and red clover in the water for 15 minutes. Strain, and reduce the liquid to 1 cup by simmering, if necessary. Add the sugar to the liquid and boil until you reach "hard-ball" stage (p.22).

Blood Thinning Mix for Long-Haul Travelers

INGREDIENTS
- ½ cup Apple Cider Vinegar (p.165)
- 2 tbsp. finely chopped fresh ginger root
- 1 head garlic, cloves separated, peeled, and crushed
- 2 tbsp. ground turmeric
- 3 tsp. cayenne powder

MAKES & KEEPS
Makes ½ cup. Keeps 1–2 years.

METHOD
Make an infused vinegar using all the ingredients (p.19).

Add 1 tbsp. to a large tomato juice at the start of your flight, repeating every 3 hours.

Do not use if you are taking warfarin or other blood-thinning drugs.

Antiseptic Hand Sanitizer

For times when you cannot wash your hands or want to give them an extra hygiene zap.

INGREDIENTS

- ¼ cup water, boiled or distilled
- 2 tsp. aloe vera gel
- 2 tbsp. distilled witch hazel

Essential oils:
- 15 drops lavender
- 15 drops tea tree
- 7 drops thyme
- oil from 2 (400 IU) vitamin E capsules (optional)

MAKES & KEEPS
Makes just under ½ cup.
Keeps 1 month.

METHOD
Mix all the ingredients together. Decant the liquid into a pocket-size spray bottle to use.

Spray directly onto hands only. Rub all over as if washing them.

Air-Con Shield

This will help prevent you from picking up your fellow passengers' bugs.

INGREDIENTS
Essential oils:
- 50 drops/½ tsp. thyme
- 100 drops/1 tsp. tea tree
- 100 drops/1 tsp. lavender

MAKES & KEEPS
Makes 2½ tsp.
Keeps at least 2 years.

METHOD
Mix the essential oils together.

Sprinkle a few drops onto a tissue or cotton ball. Wipe around the air vent above your seat (and the neighboring seats if you can) in the plane.

Mosquito Spray

Courtesy of Dedj Leibbrandt

One mosquito spray may work for one person but not another because of the way the herbs and oils mix with our own scent to create a new smell.

INGREDIENTS

- ⅔ cup distilled witch hazel
- 6 tbsp. + 2 tsp./100ml mugwort tincture (pp.18–19)

Essential oils:
- 17 drops lavender
- 17 drops thyme
- 17 drops peppermint
- 35 drops lemongrass
- 15 drops citronella
- 1 tsp. emulsifier (optional)

MAKES & KEEPS
Makes 1 cup.
Keeps 2 years.

METHOD
Simply mix the ingredients together and decant into a spray bottle. If you choose not to use an emulsifier, just shake well before each use.

Shake well before use. Apply to the skin as needed to deter mosquitoes.

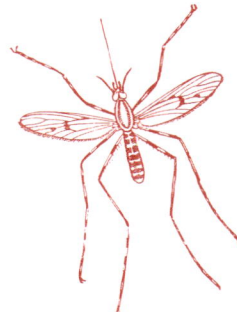

Biting Insect Repellent

Courtesy of Michael Vertolli

This will deter mosquitoes, black flies, deer flies, horse flies, fleas, and ticks. For ants, spray it for a few days at the point where they are entering the house. You can spray it on pets' bedding, but not directly on to pets.

INGREDIENTS

- 3 tbsp. + 1½ tsp. water
- 2 tbsp. + 1½ tsp. vodka
- 1 tsp. pure vegetable glycerin

Essential oils:
- 10 drops sweet basil
- 10 drops catnip
- 10 drops lavender
- 10 drops fir
- 10 drops pine
- 10 drops citronella
- 10 drops lemon or lemongrass
- 5 drops cedar
- 5 drops patchouli

MAKES & KEEPS

Makes just under ½ cup.
Keeps indefinitely.

METHOD

Mix all the ingredients together well and store in a spray bottle for ease of use.

Shake well before use. Spray on exposed areas, then spread the repellent around with your hands to make sure the entire surface of your skin is coated. Avoid contact with your eyes—to apply to face, spray your hands and rub it in carefully. If it gets into your eyes, rinse well with water.

Reapply as needed; the repellent will last for several hours.

Bug-Busting Mix for Vacation Stomaches

Take this herbal remedy alongside plain probiotic organic yogurt (or a probiotic capsule of "friendly bacteria") to help protect you from stomach bugs while traveling.

Please note that this recipe is NOT a substitute for eating and drinking sensibly — in certain countries, that means being particularly careful about water and food.

INGREDIENTS

Dried ground herbs:
- ¼ cup. fennel or cardamom
- 3 tbsp. bayberry root
- 3 tbsp. cinnamon powder
- 2 tbsp. cloves

- 10 drops thyme essential oil
- just over ¾ cup Apple Cider Vinegar (p.165)
- 3 tbsp. honey

MAKES & KEEPS

Makes 1¼ cups.
Keeps 6–12 months.

METHOD

Mix all the ingredients together well and put into a strong, wide-mouth plastic bottle for traveling. Shake or stir before use.

Take 2 tsp. daily in a little water, mixed with the freshly squeezed juice of ½ lemon, if desired.

— *Tip* —

IF YOU FEEL YOU HAVE EATEN OR DRUNK SOMETHING UNWISELY, TAKE AN EXTRA DOSE OF THE BUG-BUSTING MIX THAT DAY AND THE FOLLOWING DAY.

"Lemon Sherbet" Rehydration Remedy

It's important to drink water frequently throughout the day while you're traveling, especially in hotter climes. If you feel dehydrated, this simple recipe can help replenish your body's fluids.

INGREDIENTS
- 1 quart boiled water
- 8 tsp. sugar
- 1 tsp. salt
- grated zest and juice of 1 lemon

MAKES & KEEPS
Makes 1 quart. Drink within 2 days.

METHOD
Dissolve the sugar and salt in the water. Add the lemon. Sip often over 1–2 days to replace fluids lost by diarrhea, vomiting, or fever.

Diarrhea Stopper

Always consult a qualified healthcare practitioner if symptoms persist or are severe, especially in young children who can get dehydrated quickly.

INGREDIENTS
Dried herbs:
- 1 tbsp. green tea
- 1 tbsp. agrimony
- 2 tsp. bayberry (or yellow root)
- 2 tsp. oak bark
- 2 tsp. ground cinnamon

MAKES & KEEPS
Makes ¾-oz. herb mixture (about 4 doses). Keeps 1 year.

METHOD
Grind the herbs to powder. Mix well and store in an airtight container.

Make the tea, using 1 tbsp. mixture per mug of boiling water. Let cool and drink ½ tea cup up to 6 times in a day.

Antimalaria Mix

I carry this mix with me whenever I'm traveling to a malaria area, because these herbs can help protect against this serious disease.

INGREDIENTS
Tinctures (pp.18–19):
- ½ cup/120ml sweet wormwood
- ¼ cup/60ml bayberry

MAKES & KEEPS
Makes ¾ cup.
Keeps 2 years.

METHOD
Simply mix the tinctures together in a bottle and store.

Take 1 tsp. 3 times daily if you are in an area where malaria is active. Continue to take the mixture 1 tsp. 3 times daily for 1–2 weeks after you leave the danger area.

Caution

Malaria is a potentially life-threatening illness and precautions should always be taken when traveling to countries where it is prevalent. Always consult a health practitioner and research the subject thoroughly before traveling.

Allopathic physicians recommend taking a course of medicines to prevent malaria, though most herbalists will opt for natural alternatives. While it's possible to take both medicines and herbal treatments together, it's essential you check with your health practitioner before doing so. It's also important to note that no medicine or herb plan offers guaranteed protection against malaria. Always be vigilant against mosquitoes. Cover up and use nets and repellents as your first line of defense.

KITCHEN PHARMACY

Herbalism is a holistic form of healing that recognizes the close and vital links between body, mind, and spirit. All three elements need to be kept in harmony and balance, because all are essential to our well-being. Spirit is the most difficult concept for many Westerners; the best explanation I've heard is from plant spirit medicine expert Eliot Cowan, which I described in my book *Holistic Anatomy* (2010):

"If you think of all the movements your body makes in an hour, then compare that to where your mind goes in the same time, you can see that the mind is way faster than the body ... the mind is simply too fast for the body to grasp. Well, your spirit is to your mind what your mind is to your body—so far beyond the mind that the mind can only now and then get a glimpse of it. Yet many of us have experiences where we come close to feeling our 'spirit': highs, peak experiences, moments of deep peace, deep joy and connection, serendipity."

In treating the "whole person," herbalism acknowledges that stresses and imbalances in the body will have an effect on the mind and spirit, and vice versa.

Fortunately, Nature offers a vast medicine chest of remedies for all kinds of ailments, disorders, and diseases, upon which we can all draw. Here follows a selection of recipes for various problems of the body, mind, and spirit.

Most of these recipes use weights for dried herb amounts, because for medicines accuracy is particularly important. Many recipes also contain tinctures or mixtures of tinctures; these can be bought from a store, or made following the method in Key Preservation Techniques (pp.18–19).

With all of these recipes, consult your healthcare practitioner if symptoms persist or worsen. Conditions mentioned here may be transient or superficial, but in some cases they may be a sign of more serious illness, and lingering symptoms should always be investigated.

A note on doses

Adults

The recipes in this book all provide adult doses, as standard.

The standard dose of 1 tsp./5ml of tincture 3 times daily works well for chronic conditions; acute conditions (infections, for example) could warrant up to twice this amount over a shorter period.

See the advice on p.24 if you are pregnant, breastfeeding, or have a serious or long-lasting health condition.

Children

As a general rule, children from ages 5 to 12 are given ¼ to ½ an adult dose. From ages 12 and up, they can be given an adult dose. That said, common sense should always prevail—some children are small for their age, some are big—and doses can be adjusted accordingly. It is good to use the minimal dose you need to get the desired effect.

Babies

Babies and young children 1–5 years old should not be given tinctures. However, 1–5 tsp. of tea or decoction can be given; 1½ tsp. of syrups. At the time of writing this book, it is advisable not to give honey to babies under one year old.

Hot Stuff Circulation Stimulant

Feel warmer within minutes as these herbs zap round your bloodstream.

INGREDIENTS

Tinctures (pp.18–19):
- 2 tsp./10ml cayenne (p.156, Hot Cayenne Tincture)
- 2 tsp./10ml ginger
- 4 tsp./20ml prickly ash
- 4 tsp./20ml yarrow
- 4 tsp./20ml gingko
- 4 tsp./20ml hawthorn (p.75, Mother of the Heart Tincture)

MAKES & KEEPS

Makes just under ½ cup.
Keeps at least 3 years.

METHOD

Simply mix the tinctures together in a bottle.

Take ¼–½ tsp. in warm water every 3–4 hours as it is needed.

Horse Chestnut & Broom Varicose Vein Lotion

This effective lotion is made in the form of a liniment (p.20), so it is easy to rub in over large areas.

INGREDIENTS

- 3 tbsp. + 1 tsp. infused oil of broom tops (made with 2 tbsp. broom tops to ¼ cup + 2 tsp. of olive oil, p.20)
- 3 tbsp. + 1 tsp./50ml tincture of horse chestnut seeds (pp.18–19)

Essential oils:
- 20 drops rosemary
- 20 drops cypress

MAKES & KEEPS

Makes just under ½ cup.
Keeps at least 1 year.

METHOD

Mix all the ingredients together in a bottle.

Shake before use. Apply twice daily, massaging a small amount into the legs from ankles upward.

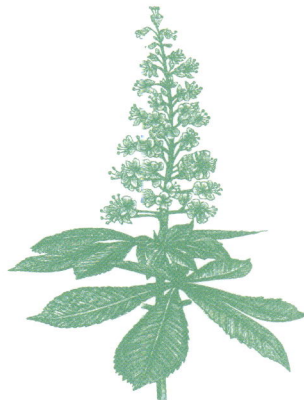

Vein-Building Complex

Courtesy of Louise Idoux

Take internally to back up external treatment of varicose veins.

INGREDIENTS
Tinctures (pp.18–19):
- 2 tbsp./30ml horse chestnut seeds
- 5 tsp./25ml butcher's broom
- 2 tsp./10ml bilberry
- 2 tsp./10ml gingko
- 5 tsp./25ml buckwheat (made using leaves and flowers)

MAKES & KEEPS
Makes just under ½ cup.
Keeps 2–3 years.

METHOD
Take ½–1 tsp. 3 times daily in a little water.

Sinusitis & Infected Teeth Mix

Courtesy of Louise Idoux

A medicine to take internally to help fight infection.

INGREDIENTS
Tinctures (pp.18–19):
- 2 tsp./10ml fresh garlic
- 2 tbsp. + 2 tsp./40ml echinacea
- 2 tsp./10ml wild indigo
- 1 tsp./5ml goldenseal
- 1 tbsp./15ml myrrh
- 4 tsp./20ml Pau d'arco

MAKES & KEEPS
Makes just under ½ cup.
Keeps indefinitely.

METHOD
Mix the tinctures and bottle.

Take 1 tsp. 3–5 times daily in a little water.

Heart & Blood Pressure Tea

Courtesy of Steve Kippax

Hawthorn helps to improve the efficiency of the heart as a muscle without increasing the oxygen used. Yarrow helps as a mild diuretic and by reducing blood pressure (you will need to take the tea for at least 6–8 weeks to experience this effect). Lime flowers are good as a relaxant, specifically affecting the heart.

INGREDIENTS
Equal parts of the following dried herbs:
- hawthorn flowering tops
- yarrow
- lime flowers

KEEPS
Keeps 1 year.

METHOD
Infuse 1 generous tsp. of the dried herbs in a mug of water for 15 minutes. Drink 3 times daily.

If one or other symptom is prevalent, then one or more of the herbs can be increased, up to double the original quantity.

— Variation —

IF YOU ADD AN EQUAL AMOUNT OF RED SAGE (DAN SHEN), THEN THE TEA MAY ALSO BE OF BENEFIT FOR CHEST PAIN/ ANGINA-TYPE SYMPTOMS. BUT AN IMPORTANT NOTE: IF YOU ARE TAKING WARFARIN OR OTHER PRESCRIPTION BLOOD-THINNING MEDICATIONS, YOU MUST CONSULT AN HERBALIST, BECAUSE THIS FORM OF SAGE CAN POTENTIATE THE MEDICINES AND THUS THE DOSAGE MAY NEED REVIEW. OTHER HERBS CAN ALSO BE OF BENEFIT FOR CARDIAC SYMPTOMS, BUT THEY ARE ONLY AVAILABLE FROM A QUALIFIED HERBALIST.

Bright Eyes Wash

This strong infusion is an effective eye wash for eye infections and sore eyes.

INGREDIENTS
Dried herbs:
- ½ oz. marigold
- ½ oz. eyebright
- ½ oz. chickweed
- ½ oz. coarsely ground Oregon grape root
- ½ oz. cornflowers

MAKES & KEEPS
Makes 2½-oz. herb mixture, enough for 15 uses.
Keeps 1–2 years in dry form. Once made up, use the same day.

METHOD
Mix the herbs together.

Infuse 1 generous tbsp. in 1 cup boiling water. Let cool, then strain carefully through cheesecloth or a thin cloth.

Wash the eyes 2–3 times daily using a sterile eye bath. Wash the eye bath well between each eye. Keep the eye wash covered between uses.

Caution
Always consult a healthcare professional for any eye problem.

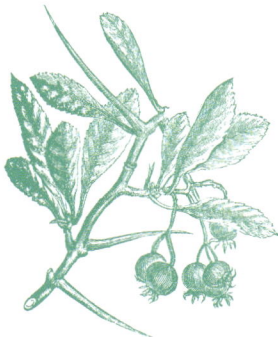

Sage & Thyme Gargle

A simple, classic gargle mixture for sore throats and warding off colds.

INGREDIENTS
- 2 cups boiling water
- 1 oz. sage leaves, dried or fresh
- 4 drops thyme essential oil

MAKES & KEEPS
Makes about 2 cups—enough for 10 gargles.
Keeps 3 days in the refrigerator.

METHOD
Pour boiling water onto the sage and let sit until lukewarm. Strain and press through cheesecloth or a thin cloth to get a dark, strong infusion. Add the essential oil and bottle.

Shake well before use, then gargle with about 3 tbsp. Repeat every hour in acute cases, otherwise use 3 times daily.

Coltsfoot Expectorant Honey

INGREDIENTS
- 1 large handful of coltsfoot flowers
- 2 cups water
- 1 cup honey

MAKES & KEEPS
Makes 2 cups.
Keeps 1 year unopened. Once open, store in the refrigerator and use within 1 month.

METHOD
Decoct the flowers in water (p.15). Simmer uncovered to reduce to 1 cup of liquid. Strain and add an equal amount of honey.

Gently heat the mixture for a few minutes to dissolve the honey. Remove from the heat and pour into bottles.

Take 1 tsp. 2–4 times daily for a cough.

Sinus-Clearing Inhalation

INGREDIENTS
- 2 cups water, almost boiling
- 1 tsp./5ml benzoin tincture (Friar's Balsam)

Essential oils:
- 1 drop thyme
- 1 drop eucalyptus
- 1 drop lavender

MAKES & KEEPS
Makes 2 cups.
Use immediately.

METHOD
Put the ingredients into a large bowl. Carefully cover your head and the bowl with a towel to trap the steam inside. Inhale through the nose until there is no more steam.

Repeat every 4 hours as required.

— Tip —

FRIAR'S BALSAM TINCTURE LEAVES A RESIDUE OF RESIN ON THE SIDE OF THE CONTAINER THAT IS HARD TO WASH OFF. KEEP A CONTAINER ASIDE FOR ONLY FRIAR'S BALSAM USE, UNLESS YOU LIKE A LOT OF SCRUBBING!

Vapor Rub

Courtesy of Neil Williams

Rub into chest and neck to help relieve breathing and fight chest infections.

INGREDIENTS
- just over ⅓ cup + 2 tbsp. olive oil
- 1 tbsp. grated beeswax

Essential oils:
- 60 drops eucalyptus
- 60 drops pine
- 60 drops peppermint
- 60 drops cajeput
- 60 drops cedarwood

MAKES & KEEPS
Makes just under ½ cup.
Keeps 1 year.

METHOD
Gently melt the beeswax into the olive oil in a double boiler or water bath. Let the mixture cool for 5 minutes, then add the essential oils and pour into one or more jars.

Use sparingly.

Caution

Do not use on children under 2 years. Keep away from the eyes and delicate tissues.

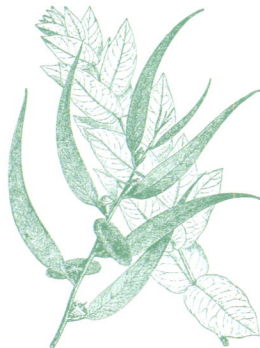

Truly Tasty Cough Mixture

Courtesy of Geoff Edwards

INGREDIENTS
Dried herbs:
- ¾ oz. coltsfoot
- ¾ oz. Irish moss
- ¾ oz. licorice root
- ½ oz. thyme
- ½ oz. elecampane
- ½ oz. white horehound

- 1½ quarts water
- 1¼ oz. ground marshmallow root
- 36 oz. honey

Essential oils:
- 60 drops eucalyptus
- 60 drops anise seed
- 30 drops peppermint

- ½ tsp. quillea fluid extract (p.18)

MAKES & KEEPS
Makes about 2 quarts.
Keeps 1 year.

METHOD
Simmer all the dried herbs except for the marshmallow root in the water for 30 minutes, then strain. Measure the liquid and make up the volume to 5¼ cups (add more water or reduce the liquid further, as required).

Meanwhile, make a smooth paste from the marshmallow with a little water. Then add more water to make up to 2 cups.

Add to the herbal mix in the saucepan with the honey. Bring to a boil and simmer briskly for 5 minutes. Remove from the heat and cool.

You should have about 2 quarts of liquid. Separately, mix together the essential oils and quillea tincture (this emulsifies the essential oils so they do not separate), then add it to the rest.

Take 1–2 tsp. 3–4 times daily, neat or with a little warm water.

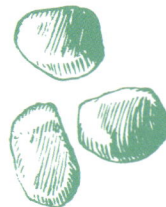

Rose Hip, Hawthorn & Pine Throat Lozenges

INGREDIENTS
- 3 generous handfuls of fresh rose hips
- 2 generous handfuls of fresh hawthorn berries
- up to 1½ cups golden syrup or light corn syrup
- up to 2½ cups sugar
- 3 tbsp. + 1 tsp./50ml pine tincture (pp.18–19)
- 20 drops lemon essential oil

YOU WILL NEED
· CANDY MOLDS OR BAKING SHEET (P.22)

MAKES & KEEPS
Makes 100 or so lozenges.
Keeps up to 6 weeks in a container in the refrigerator.

METHOD
Collect your berries, and immediately decoct in enough water to cover (p.15), covered, for 10 minutes. Let cool. Mash up the mixture a little, then strain through a double layer of cheesecloth. Mix this liquid (probably about 1⅔ cups) with equal amounts of both sugar and golden or corn syrup.

Make into candies (pp.21–22), stirring in the pine tincture and lemon essential oil just before pouring the mixture into molds.

Lichen, Coltsfoot & Thyme Cough Candies

INGREDIENTS
- 2 handfuls of lung lichen
- 2 cups water
- up to 2 cups sugar
- up to 1¼ cups golden syrup or light corn syrup
- 3 tbsp. + 1 tsp./50ml coltsfoot tincture (pp.18–19)
- 20 drops thyme essential oil

YOU WILL NEED
· CANDY MOLDS

MAKES & KEEPS
Makes 100–200 small hard candies.
Keeps up to 6 weeks.

METHOD
Make a decoction by bringing the lichen and water to a boil (p.15), then simmering for 10 minutes with the lid on. Let the mixture sit to cool, then strain.

Mix this liquid (about 1⅔ cups) with equal amounts of sugar and golden or corn syrup. Make into candies (pp.21–22), stirring in the coltsfoot tincture and thyme essential oil just before pouring the mixture into molds.

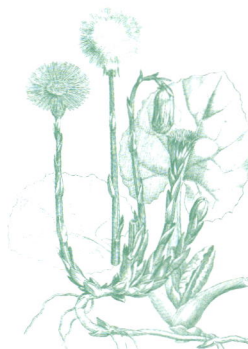

Antinausea Tea

If you can keep it down, this can help with nausea.

INGREDIENTS
Dried herbs:
- 1 oz. chamomile
- 1 oz. peppermint
- 1 oz. roughly ground root ginger

MAKES & KEEPS
Makes 3-oz. herb mixture.
Keeps at least 1 year.

METHOD
Mix the herbs together and store in a jar.

Make the tea using 1 tsp. per mug, infused for 5 minutes.

Take 4–5 times daily.

Antinausea Suppositories

Courtesy of Dedj Leibbrandt

Use these when you feel too nauseous to take anything by mouth. The cocoa butter melts and releases the essential oils; these enter the bloodstream and exert their medicinal effect.

INGREDIENTS
- 4 tsp. cocoa butter

Essential oils:
- 12 drops chamomile
- 4 drops peppermint
- 4 drops lemon
- 1 drop ginger

YOU WILL NEED
· 7 (2-G) SUPPOSITORY MOLDS

MAKES & KEEPS
Makes 7 suppositories.
Keeps 3 months in the refrigerator.

METHOD
Gently warm the cocoa butter in a double boiler or water bath until melted. Mix in the essential oils, pour into molds, and put into the refrigerator to set. Once set (usually after about 30 minutes), remove from the molds and store.

Insert one into your buttocks as needed, or every 3–4 hours.

Marshmallow Water for Acid Indigestion

This is also good for coughs and catarrh.

INGREDIENTS
- 21 oz. ground dried marshmallow root (or 1 small handful of freshly dug roots)
- 2 cups cold water
- 1–2 tbsp. honey (optional; if using, manuka is the best)

MAKES & KEEPS
Makes 2 cups.
Keeps 3–4 days in the refrigerator.

METHOD
Soak the marshmallow in the water for 30 minutes. When softened, process in a blender for a few minutes until smooth. Add the honey, if using, and let sit for 4 hours. Bottle and keep in the refrigerator.

Take 2 tbsp. 3 times daily until symptoms are finished.

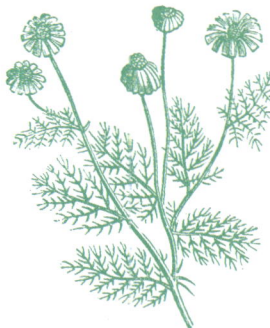

Heartburn Tea

Courtesy of Steve Kippax

This tea is great for stomach pain, heartburn, and reflux. The meadowsweet helps to reduce the inflammation in the stomach and marshmallow root coats the stomach lining with a healing coat. Licorice stops the pain and reflux associated with gastritis and heartburn.

INGREDIENTS
Dried herbs:
- **2 oz. meadowsweet**
- **2 oz. ground marshmallow root**
- **2 oz. ground licorice root**

MAKES & KEEPS
Makes 6-oz. herb mixture.
Keeps 1–2 years.

METHOD
Mix the dried herbs together and store.

Take 1 generous tsp. of the dried herbs infused in a mug of hot water for 15 minutes 3–4 times daily.

Gas-Reducing Syrup

For promoting good digestion and liver function.

INGREDIENTS
- **1 handful of fresh angelica root, coarsely chopped (or 2 oz. dried)**
- **1 quart water**
- **1 (12-oz.) jar of honey**
- **juice of 2 lemons**

MAKES & KEEPS
Makes 22 fl. oz.
Keeps up to 1 year in the refrigerator.

METHOD
Simmer the angelica for 2½ hours in the water. Strain and reduce to 1¼ cups of liquid. Add the honey and lemon juice. Gently warm and stir to dissolve the honey, then pour into bottles, tightening the lids when cool.

Take 1 tsp. 1–3 times daily as required.

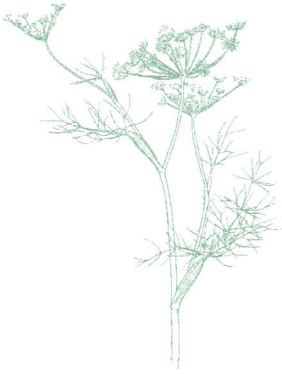

Irritable Bowel Tincture Mix

Courtesy of Louise Idoux

INGREDIENTS
Tinctures (pp.18–19):
- **3 tbsp. + 1 tsp./50ml chamomile**
- **2 tsp./10ml cardamom**
- **1 tbsp./15ml fennel**
- **2 tsp./10ml wild yam**
- **2 tsp./10ml cramp bark**

MAKES & KEEPS
Makes just under ½ cup.
Keeps 2–3 years.

METHOD
Simply mix and bottle.

Take 1 tsp. in warm water 3 times daily.

Antispasmodic Drops

Courtesy of Dedj Leibbrandt

A practitioner–level remedy for intestinal spasm consisting of a blend of tinctures. Measure using a millimeter measure—accuracy is important.

INGREDIENTS
Tinctures (pp.18–19):
- 10ml cramp bark (fluid extract if possible, p.18)
- 4ml pasqueflower
- 4ml yellow jasmine
- 2ml henbane

MAKES & KEEPS
Makes 20 ml.
Keeps 2–3 years.

METHOD
Mix the tinctures together in a dropper bottle.

Take 10 drops in a little water every hour until spasms ease. Do not exceed 10 doses in 24 hours (see box below).

Always seek your healthcare practitioner's advice to determine the cause of pain.

Caution

Henbane and yellow jasmine are strong herbs that are harmful in large doses. Very small amounts are used by herbal practitioners: a maximum of 5 ml—1 tsp.—per week (equal to 5 drops taken 3 times daily). In some countries, only herbal practitioners are permitted to purchase these plants.

Worm Suppositories

Courtesy of Dedj Leibbrandt

For greatest success, use these alongside the Intestinal Parasite Treatment (p.104).

INGREDIENTS
- 4 tsp. cocoa butter

Essential oils:
- 10 drops vetiver
- 10 drops oregano
- 5 drops cloves
- 5 drops roman chamomile

YOU WILL NEED
· 7 (2-G) SUPPOSITORY MOLDS

MAKES & KEEPS
Makes 7 suppositories.
Keeps 3 months in the refrigerator.

METHOD
Gently melt the cocoa butter in a double boiler or water bath. Mix in the essential oils and pour into the molds.

Insert 1 into your buttocks evening and morning for 4 days either side of the new moon and full moon (when worms are most active).

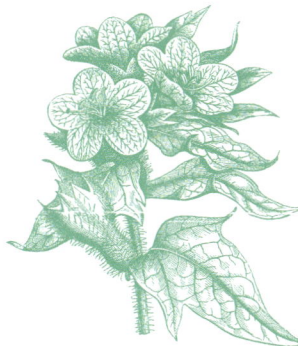

Intestinal Parasite Treatment

Use these alongside the Worm Suppositories (p.103) for best effect.

INGREDIENTS

Tinctures (pp.18–19):
- 3 tbsp. + 1 tsp./50ml cloves
- 3 tbsp. + 1 tsp./50ml bayberry
- 3 tbsp. + 1 tsp./50ml wormwood
- 3 tbsp. + 1 tsp./50ml black walnut

To administer:
- 2 tsp. flaxseeds
- 1 handful of pumpkin seeds (approx. 20)

MAKES & KEEPS

Makes just over ¾ cup.
Keeps at least 2 years.

METHOD

Mix the tinctures together. Put 2 tsp. of the tincture mix in just over ¾ cup water.

To administer, grind the flaxseeds and mix them with the drink. Eat the pumpkin seeds, washing them down with the drink.

Do this once daily for 3 weeks. Let sit for 1 week, then repeat for 2 weeks.

— Tip —

IF YOU CAN GET HOLD
OF THEM, FRESH PAPAYAS CAN
ALSO BE USED TO TREAT WORMS.
TAKE 2 TSP. FRESH PAPAYA SEEDS
EVERY DAY FOR 3 WEEKS.
CHEW THEM WELL.

Bowel Cleanse

Best used alongside a detox diet. If possible, eat a whole-food diet for at least 2–3 weeks before starting to take this mixture.

INGREDIENTS

Dried ground herbs:
- 2 oz. yellow dock root
- 2 oz. turkey rhubarb root
- 2 oz. plantain leaves
- 2 oz. Californian buckthorn bark
- 2 oz. barberry bark

MAKES & KEEPS

Makes 10 oz. (enough for 3 weeks).
Keeps 1 year.

Fresh:
- 2 tbsp. aloe vera gel
- 2-inch piece fresh ginger root, grated
- 4 garlic cloves, finely chopped
- 1 quart apple juice
- 2 tsp. psyllium husks

MAKES & KEEPS

Makes 1 day's dose.
Use fresh.

METHOD

Thoroughly mix together the ground herbs.

Take 4 tsp. of the mixture and add the aloe, ginger, garlic, and apple juice. Mix well.

Take in the morning, adding the psyllium husks to the last one-quarter of the liquid.

Drink daily for 3 weeks.

Do not give to children under 12 without professional advice.

Milk Thistle Liver Protector

Milk thistle has the ability to protect the liver from toxins, as well as to support a damaged liver while it regenerates.

INGREDIENTS
- 4 oz. milk thistle seeds, dried and ground

MAKES & KEEPS
Makes 50–60 doses.
Keeps 1 year.

METHOD
Take 1 tsp. stirred into ½ mug of warm water 1–2 times daily.

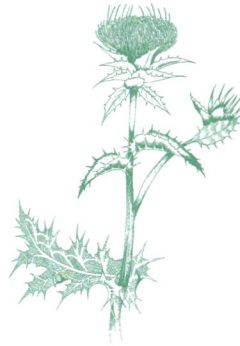

Bentonite Clay Cleanser

Clay is extremely absorbent, so it draws toxic substances. In the bowel, it will draw all kinds of toxins and help to eliminate them from the body.

INGREDIENTS
- 1 tsp. clay
- 1 mug of chamomile tea (p.15)

MAKES & KEEPS
Makes 1 dose.
Drink immediately.

METHOD
Soak the clay in the chamomile tea for the day. Take on an empty stomach before bed.

Take daily for 3 weeks, then have a break for at least a week.

Coconut Liver Blast

This mixture is a good general boost for the liver, helpful alongside a detox diet. The mix is taken with coconut oil, which has been found to protect the liver from toxins.

INGREDIENTS
Dried ground herbs:
- 3 oz. dandelion leaves
- 3 oz. milk thistle seeds
- 3 oz. angelica archangelica root
- 1 (12-oz.) jar of virgin coconut oil

MAKES & KEEPS
Makes 21 oz.
Keeps at least 6 months.

METHOD
Gently melt the coconut oil in the jar in a double boiler or water bath and thoroughly mix in the herbs. Pour into a large jar and let set in a cool place for 30–60 minutes.

Take 1 tbsp. 1–2 times daily.

Cystitis Tea

INGREDIENTS
Dried herbs:
- I oz. buchu leaves
- I oz. plantain leaves
- I oz. yarrow flowering tops
- I oz. marshmallow leaves

MAKES & KEEPS
Makes 4-oz. herb mixture.
Keeps I–2 years.

METHOD
Mix the herbs well. Make the tea, using 2 tbsp. to I quart water (p.15).

Strain and drink over I day.

Repeat daily and continue for 5 days after the symptoms clear. Usually, the symptoms improve almost immediately, but if you stop taking the tea too soon, they will come back—the infection needs to be thoroughly cleared.

— *Tip* —

FOR CYSTITIS PREVENTION,
TAKE I MUG OF CYSTITIS TEA,
MADE FROM I TSP. PER MUG,
DAILY.

Cystitis Routine

Courtesy of Dedj Leibbrandt

INGREDIENTS
Tinctures (pp.18–19):
- ½ cup + 2 tbsp./150ml cornsilk
- ¼ cup + I tbsp./75ml buchu
- ¼ cup + I tbsp./75ml bearberry

MAKES & KEEPS
Makes about I¼ cups.
Keeps 2–3 years.

METHOD
Put just under ½ cup of the mixture into I quart water.

Sip it over 24 hours and repeat the next day. On days 3 and 4, put just under ¼ cup into I quart water. Sip it over 24 hours. You must complete the 4-day course.

Do not give to children under 12.

Caution

If you don't feel better after the first 24 hours of this treatment, then you need antibiotics; see your doctor. Bladder infections must be treated quickly, because they can track up to the kidneys with serious consequences.

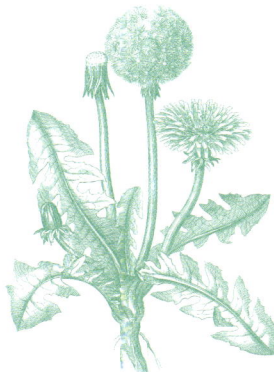

Waterfall Smoothie

Courtesy of Anne McIntyre

To help treat the retention of premenstrual fluid.

INGREDIENTS
⅓ cup of the following fresh herbs:
- wild celery leaves
- dandelion leaves
- fennel leaves and/or seeds
- cilantro leaves and/or coriander seeds
- nasturtium leaves and flowers
- parsley leaves
- 1 bunch of celery, chopped
- 1 cucumber, chopped

YOU WILL NEED
· A BLENDER

MAKES & KEEPS
Makes 1 serving.
Drink immediately.

METHOD
Blend all the ingredients until smooth.

Drink the smoothie for breakfast first thing in the morning, and repeat throughout the day as often as desired. Continue over a few days, or over a few weeks if the problem is chronic.

Incontinence Tea

Helps to strengthen the bladder.

INGREDIENTS
Dried herbs:
- 1 oz. horsetail
- 1 oz. couchgrass
- 1 oz. shepherd's purse
- 1 oz. borage
- 1 oz. marshmallow leaves

MAKES & KEEPS
Makes 5-oz. tea mix.
Keeps 1–2 years.

METHOD
Make the tea, using 2 tsp. per mug (p.15).

Drink 2–3 cups daily.

Ladies' Lovelies

Courtesy of Sensory Solutions

These protective, nurturing, and balancing drops help to support women of any age. They help with traumatic pregnancy and birth experiences and other female gynecological issues, such as difficult menstruation, problems in conceiving, and menopause.

INGREDIENTS

- 2 tbsp./30ml raspberry leaf tincture (pp.18–19)
- 2 tbsp./30ml lady's mantle tincture (pp.18–19)
- 2 tbsp. nettle syrup (pp.21–22)

MAKES & KEEPS

Makes just over ⅓ cup.
Keeps at least a year.

METHOD

Mix the ingredients together in a dropper bottle.

Take 5–10 drops 3–6 times daily as required.

Nettle Syrup

Delicious and rich in minerals and vitamin C.

INGREDIENTS

- 3 cups water
- 2 oz. dried nettles (or 2 cups fresh)
- 2 cups sugar (I prefer brown)

MAKES & KEEPS

Makes about 3 cups
Keeps 3–12 months.

METHOD

Bring the water and nettles to a boil. Simmer for 10 minutes with the lid on. Let steep for 3–4 hours, then strain.

Reduce the liquid to 2 cups. Add the sugar and boil for an additional 4–5 minutes, then pour into bottles.

Take 1-2 tsp. daily as a mineral-rich syrup or use diluted with carbonated water as a beverage.

PMS Chocolates

These bittersweet chocolates contain a daily dose of PMS-busting herbs.

INGREDIENTS

- ½ cup cocoa butter
- ½ cup coconut oil
- 1 cup raw chocolate powder
- 2 tsp. ground chasteberry (this herb tastes bitter)
- ⅓ oz. dried and ground lady's mantle
- about 2 tbsp. honey, agave syrup, or maple syrup, to taste
- 1 handful of raspberries, dried or fresh
- 1 handful of chopped nuts
- 2 drops rose otto essential oil

YOU WILL NEED

· SMALL MOLDS, SUCH AS ICE CUBE TRAYS

MAKES & KEEPS

Makes 40 ice cube-size chocolates.
Keeps 2–3 months in the freezer.

METHOD

Put all ingredients except the honey/syrup, raspberries, nuts, and rose otto essential oil into a double boiler or water bath. Melt the butter over gentle heat, stirring constantly. Do not overheat. Add the honey/syrup to taste, and the raspberries and nuts, continuing to stir.

When you are satisfied with the sweetness, remove from the heat. Stir in the rose otto essential oil and pour into the molds. (Put about 1 tbsp. into each.)

Let set in the refrigerator for 30–60 minutes.

Eat 1 chocolate daily to help balance your hormones. You may use this remedy for 3–12 months. Don't stop and start; take continuously as the chasteberry works best that way.

When the PMS is most acute and you want to eat more chocolates, switch to No Stress Raw Chocolates (opposite).

No Stress Raw Chocolates

INGREDIENTS
- ½ cup cocoa butter
- ½ cup coconut oil
- I cup raw chocolate powder
- 2 tbsp. ground valerian
- 4 tbsp. dried ground passionflower
- 2 tbsp. dried rose petals, broken into small pieces
- I–2 tbsp. honey, agave syrup, or maple syrup
- 2 drops rose otto essential oil
- 2 tbsp. cocoa nibs
- 2 tbsp. shelled hemp seeds

YOU WILL NEED
· SMALL MOLDS, SUCH AS ICE CUBE TRAYS

MAKES & KEEPS
Makes 40 ice cube-size chocolates.
Keeps 3 months in the freezer.

METHOD
Put all ingredients except the honey/syrup, rose otto essential oil, cocoa nibs, and hemp seeds into a double boiler or water bath. Melt the cocoa butter over gentle heat, stirring constantly. Do not overheat. Add the honey/syrup to taste, continuing to stir.

When you are satisfied with the sweetness, remove from the heat. Stir in the rose otto essential oil, nibs, and seeds, then pour it into the molds. (Put about I tbsp. into each.)

Eat up to 4–5 daily in the days leading up to your period, or at any other stressful time.

Period Pain Chocolates

INGREDIENTS
- ½ cup cocoa butter
- ½ cup coconut oil
- I cup raw chocolate powder
- 4 tsp. ground cinnamon
- 4 tsp. dried ground cramp bark
- 5 tsp. skullcap
- I–2 tbsp. honey, agave syrup or maple syrup
- ¼ cup cocoa nibs, shelled hemp seeds, or chopped nuts

YOU WILL NEED
· SMALL MOLDS, SUCH AS ICE CUBE TRAYS

MAKES & KEEPS
Makes 40 ice cube-size chocolates.
Keeps 3 months in the freezer.

METHOD
Put all ingredients except the honey/syrup and nibs/seeds/nuts into a double boiler or water bath. Melt the cocoa butter over gentle heat, stirring constantly. Do not overheat. Add the honey/syrup to taste, continuing to stir.

When you are satisfied with the sweetness, remove from the heat, add the nibs/seeds/nuts, and pour it into the molds. (Put about I tbsp. into each.)

Eat I chocolate every 20 minutes until period pain has eased, then I every 3 hours.

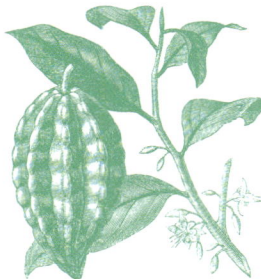

Period Pain Tea

Courtesy of Anne McIntyre

INGREDIENTS
Dried herbs:

- 2 oz. rose
- 2 oz. motherwort
- 2 oz. lady's mantle
- 2 oz. chamomile
- 2 oz. clary sage

MAKES & KEEPS
Makes 10-oz. herb mixture
(enough for 10 days).
Keeps 1 year.

METHOD
Mix the herbs together. Put 2 oz. of the herb mix into a teapot. Pour 1 quart boiling water over the herbs and infuse for 10–15 minutes.

Drink 1 mug 3 times daily throughout the month.

On the first day of the period, or whenever there is the most discomfort, drink throughout the day as needed, up to 6 mugs.

Cream for Vaginal Thrush

This versatile cream can also be used for men's thrush and for oral thrush.

INGREDIENTS

- ¼ cup Heal-All Marigold Cream (p.81)

Essential oils:
- 6 drops tea tree
- 6 drops niaouli
- 6 drops palmarosa
- 2 drops oregano

MAKES & KEEPS
Makes ¼ cup.
Keeps at least 6 months in the refrigerator.

METHOD
Mix the marigold cream and essential oils together.

Apply to the affected area 1–2 times daily.

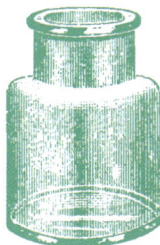

Pessaries for Thrush

Courtesy of Dedj Leibbrandt

These help to soothe itching and restore vaginal health.

INGREDIENTS
- 8 tsp. cocoa butter

Essential oils:
- 13 drops tea tree
- 13 drops niaouli
- 13 drops palmarosa
- 4 drops oregano

YOU WILL NEED
· 14 (2-G) MOLDS

MAKES & KEEPS
Makes 14 pessaries.
Keeps 3 months in the refrigerator.

METHOD
Gently warm the cocoa butter in a double boiler or water bath until melted. Mix in the essential oils and pour into the molds.

Insert 1 pessary as high as you can into the vagina 2 times daily. Lie down for 10–30 minutes after inserting.

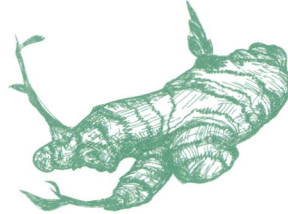

Morning Sickness Candies

INGREDIENTS
- ½ handful of chopped fresh ginger root
- 1 oz. dried black horehound (double the quantity if fresh)
- just under 2 cups water
- 2¾ cups brown sugar
- 4 tbsp. butter (optional)

YOU WILL NEED
· CANDY MOLDS

MAKES & KEEPS
Makes about 100 hard candies.
Keeps 4–6 weeks in a container in the refrigerator.

METHOD
Boil the ginger and horehound in water for 20 minutes. Strain and make the candies (pp.21–22).

If using butter, add it just before pouring the candy mix into the molds.

Take 4–8 candies daily, and enjoy.

FOR LABOR

These are a few remedies to assist labor. All are tinctures unless otherwise stated, which can be bought from a store or be homemade as instructed on pages 18–19. Always take tinctures by mixing them with water.

Please be aware that these remedies should only be used to assist birth where necessary, and should never be used in place of proper medical attention.

Labor Endurance Mix

To help keep up strength for labor.

INGREDIENTS
- 1 oz. dried raspberry leaves
- 1 oz. dried lady's mantle leaves
- 1 quart boiling water
- ¼ cup/50ml American ginseng tincture (pp.18–19)

MAKES & KEEPS
Makes 1 quart.
Keeps 2 days.

METHOD
Make a tea from the raspberry leaves, lady's mantle leaves, and water (p.15). Add the ginseng tincture. Sip throughout labor from the start.

Contractions Booster

To make weak contractions stronger, and to help expel the placenta.

INGREDIENTS
- golden seal tincture (pp.18–19) or dried ground root

METHOD
Take 1–2 tsp. every 1–2 hours. If using the dried form, take ½–1 tsp. Note: It tastes vile!

Relaxing Mix for Labor

This is to take during labor if contractions are too strong and painful early on.

INGREDIENTS
Tinctures (pp.18–19):
- 1 tbsp./15ml lobelia
- 2 tbsp. + 2 tsp./40ml blue cohosh
- 2 tbsp. + 2 tsp./40ml cramp bark
- 1 tsp./5ml yellow jasmine

MAKES & KEEPS
Makes just under ½ cup.
Keeps 2–3 years.

METHOD
Take 1 tsp. every 1–2 hours. If the cervix is not opening, take 1 tbsp. in a single dose.

Antihemorrhage Mix

This mixture can be used to slow any bleeding anywhere in the body.

INGREDIENTS
Tinctures (pp.18–19):
- 2 tbsp./30ml yarrow
- 2 tbsp./30ml shepherd's purse
- 2 tbsp./30ml goldenseal

MAKES & KEEPS
Makes 6 tbsp.
Keeps 2–3 years.

METHOD
Mix the tinctures together in a bottle.

Call an ambulance if medics are not already there. Take 4 tsp, followed by another 4 tsp. in 15 minutes if still bleeding.

No-Sweat Sage Tea

Particularly useful for menopausal night sweats,
sage can help any excessive sweating.

INGREDIENTS
- 3 tbsp. dried chopped sage leaves
  and flowers
- I quart boiling water

MAKES & KEEPS
Makes I quart (enough for 2 days).
Keeps up to 3 days in the refrigerator.

METHOD
Put the sage into a teapot or lidded saucepan.
Cover with the boiling water, add the lid, and
let cool. Strain and drink cold.

Take I mug 3 times daily for several weeks.

Syrupy Menopause Mix

A delicious way to take these female hormone-
boosting herbs.

INGREDIENTS
- ½ cup/120ml wild yam root tincture
  (pp.18–19)
- ½ cup/120ml red clover syrup (pp.21–22)

MAKES & KEEPS
I cup.
Keeps I year.

METHOD
Mix the tincture and syrup together and bottle.
Take ½–2 tsp. 2–3 times daily.

Note
Treatments for hormone conditions often take at
least 3 months to take full effect.

Herbal "HRT" Cream

This do-it-yourself cream is made from wild yam.
Many women swear by it to help keep menopausal
symptoms at bay.

INGREDIENTS
- 6 tbsp. + 2 tsp. evening primrose oil
- ½ cup emulsifying wax
- ¾ cup + 5 tsp. wild yam root tea (p.15)
- 6 tbsp. + 2 tsp./100ml wild yam tincture
  (pp.18–19)

Essential oils (optional):
- 20 drops jasmine
- 20 drops neroli
- 20 drops clary sage
- ½ tsp./2ml benzoin tincture
  (Friar's Balsam)

MAKES & KEEPS
Makes just under 2 cups.
Keeps up to I year.

METHOD
Make as for Comfrey Cream for Speedy Healing
(p.82), mixing in the essential oils, if using,
with the benzoin.

To use, rub I tsp. of the cream into soft skin
(inside the arms, inner thighs, belly, breasts)
1–2 times daily.

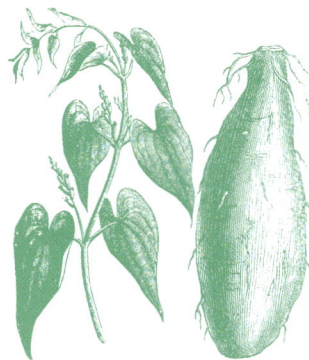

Balancing Tincture for Menopause

Courtesy of Anne McIntyre

INGREDIENTS
Dried herbs:
- 4 oz. red sage leaves
- 4 oz. motherwort
- 4 oz. lady's mantle
- 4 oz. chamomile
- 4 oz. rose petals
  (or use 9 oz. each of fresh herbs)
- 2 cups brandy or vodka

MAKES & KEEPS
Makes about 1⅔ cups/400ml tincture.
Keeps 2–3 years.

METHOD
Make a tincture from the ingredients (pp.18–19).

Take 1–2 tsp. 3 times daily in a little water.

It may take 3 weeks–3 months to benefit fully.

Tea for Dizziness

INGREDIENTS
Dried ground herbs:
- 2 oz. rosemary leaves
- 2 oz. gingko leaves
- 2 oz. wood betony leaves

MAKES & KEEPS
Makes 6-oz. herb mixture.
Keeps 1–2 years.

METHOD
Mix well and store in a jar.

Make the tea as required, using 1 tsp.
per mug (p.15).

Take 3 mugs daily.

Cramp-Relieving Tincture

Courtesy of Anthony Seifert

Helps to treat menstrual cramping and cramping due to dysentery, as well as headaches, sleeplessness, and anxiety.

INGREDIENTS
Tinctures (pp.18–19):
- 3 tbsp./45ml California poppy
- 2 tbsp./30ml silk tassel
- 1 tbsp./15ml lemon balm
- 1 tbsp./15ml Jamaican dogwood bark

MAKES & KEEPS
Makes just under ½ cup.
Keeps 2–3 years.

METHOD
Combine all the tinctures and bottle.

Take 10–30 drops up to 5 times daily until pain subsides.

Women's Balancing Tea (Swiss Style)

Courtesy of Christine Herren–Valette

This tea helps to harmonize the menstrual cycle.

INGREDIENTS
Dried ground herbs:
- 3 tbsp. yarrow
- 2 tbsp. raspberry leaf
- 2 tbsp. lady's mantle
- 2 tbsp. marigold flowers
- 5 tsp. sage

MAKES & KEEPS
Makes 1-oz. herb mixture.
Keeps 1 year.

METHOD
Mix the herbs together. Make the tea (p.15), using 1 tsp. of the herb mixture per mug of hot water.

Take 1–3 cups daily.

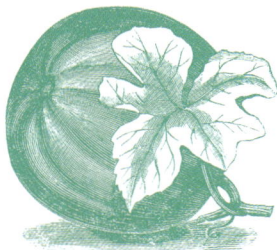

Herbal Tonic for Prostate Health

Many men experience prostate problems and can benefit from prostate-supporting herbs.

INGREDIENTS

Dried herbs:
- ½ oz. nettle root
- ½ oz. saw palmetto
- ½ oz. horsetail
- ½ oz. raspberry leaf
- ½ oz. plantain
- 1 tbsp. white cedar

- 2 cups organic Apple Cider Vinegar (p.165) or organic vodka

MAKES & KEEPS

Makes about 1⅔ cups.
Keeps 2–3 years.

METHOD

Make a tincture or infused vinegar (pp.18–19).

Take 1 tsp. 3 times daily in a little water.

— Tip —

TAKE 1–2 TBSP. PUMPKIN SEEDS
DAILY TO BOOST YOUR
ZINC LEVELS. PLENTY OF EXERCISE
WILL ALSO HELP.

Men's Reproductive Tonic

May support in treating infertility and impotence.

INGREDIENTS

Dried ground herbs:
- 2 oz. horsetail
- 2 oz. damiana
- 2 oz. ginseng

- ¾ cup pumpkin seeds
- 1 (12-oz.) jar of virgin coconut oil

MAKES & KEEPS

Makes 22 oz.
Keeps at least 1 year.

METHOD

Mix together the herbs and seeds. Separately, melt the coconut oil in a double boiler or water bath. Mix the herbs/seeds and oil together thoroughly and jar. Let set for 30–60 minutes in a cool place. Once set, store in a cool place.

Take 1 tbsp. daily.

Antianxiety Drops with Valerian & Rose

INGREDIENTS
- 1 oz. valerian root
- ½ oz. rosebuds
- 2 cups brandy
- 1 tbsp. honey

MAKES & KEEPS

Makes just under 2 cups.
Keeps 2–3 years.

METHOD

Mix all the ingredients together and put into a large jar with a lid. Let sit in a cool place for 3 weeks. Strain and bottle.

Take 5–10 drops as required, up to 6 times daily.

Herbal Antidepressant

This mix almost always lifts the spirits, without making you feel numb or interfering with painful emotions.

INGREDIENTS

Dried and powdered herbs:
- 3 oz. oat straw
- 3 oz. rosemary
- 3 oz. lemon balm
- 3 oz. St. John's wort
- 1 (12-oz.) jar of honey or pure coconut oil

MAKES & KEEPS

Makes 24 oz.
Keeps 6–12 months.

METHOD

Mix the herbs together. Warm the honey or oil and mix well with the herbs. Pour into jars.

Take 1–2 tsp. 1–3 times daily (if you feel really down, go for the higher dose of 2 tsp, then reduce it as you start to feel better).

False Solomon's Seal & Teasel for Joints

Courtesy of Matthew Wood

This acts on the carpals and tarsals and on the pelvic floor. It is also great for the small joints of the fingers if treating rheumatoid arthritis.

INGREDIENTS

Tinctures (pp.18–19):
- ¼ cup/60ml false Solomon's seal or "dragon root"
- ¼ cup/60ml teasel

MAKES & KEEPS

Makes ½ cup.
Keeps 2–3 years.

METHOD

Mix the tinctures together in a bottle.

Take 3–5 drops 3 times daily.

Solomon's Seal & Agrimony Tension Remedy

Courtesy of Matthew Wood

This remedy for tension, both psychological and physical, relaxes most people in seconds. It's made with 7 parts agrimony to 4 parts Solomon's seal.

INGREDIENTS

Tinctures (pp.18–19):
- ¾ cup + 6 tsp./210ml agrimony (but make this with 1½ handfuls of fresh agrimony and 1–2 cups good brandy, enough to cover)
- ½ cup/120ml Solomon's seal (but make this with 1½ handfuls of Solomon's seal roots—unearthed, coarsely chopped, and placed in a jar—and 2 cups vodka)

MAKES & KEEPS

Makes about 2 cups.
Keeps at least 2 years.

METHOD

Mix the tinctures together in a bottle.

Take 3–5 drops 3 times daily (or as needed).

— Tip —

PICK THE AGRIMONY LEAVES OFF THE SIDES OF THE LEADER OR MAIN STEM, SO THAT THE LATTER CAN GO ON TO FLOWERING.

SOLOMON'S SALVES

The following variations on Solomon's seal salve come from the highly regarded American herbalist Matthew Wood. All feature the infused oil of true Solomon's seal root. To make it, use 7 oz. dry plant material and enough safflower or olive oil to cover (about 1 cup; see p.20). To make each salve recipe, simply heat all the ingredients together until the beeswax has melted, stir, and pour into jars.

All these recipes make 4 full 2-oz. jars, with possibly a little left over, and keep for at least 12 months in the refrigerator.

Apply these salves liberally to sore, affected areas 1–3 times daily.

Joint-Aligning Salve

This helps to tighten loose joints and bring them back into alignment.

INGREDIENTS
- ¾ cup + 5 tsp. infused oil of true Solomon's seal (see recipe above)
- 1,600 IU vitamin E oil
- 2 tbsp. + 2 tsp. Comfrey Oil (p.80)
- 3 tbsp. grated beeswax

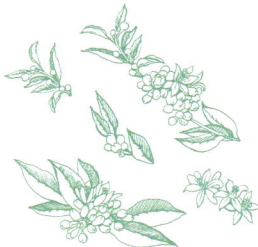

Solomon's Bad Back Salve

This muscle and joint-relaxing salve has a particular affinity with the back.

INGREDIENTS
- ¾ cup + 5 tsp. infused oil of true Solomon's seal (see recipe left)
- 1,600 IU vitamin E oil
- 2 tbsp. + 2 tsp. ginger root infused oil (p.20)
- 3 tbsp. grated beeswax

Salve for Dry Joints

Adding marshmallow seems to enhance Solomon's seal's ability to moisten and nourish the joints.

INGREDIENTS
- ¾ cup + 5 tsp. infused oil of true Solomon's seal (see recipe above left)
- 1,600 IU vitamin E oil
- 2 tbsp. + 2 tsp. marshmallow root infused oil (p.20)
- 3 tbsp. grated beeswax

Cartilage-Healing Salve

INGREDIENTS
- ¾ cup + 1 tbsp. infused oil of true Solomon's seal (see recipe above left)
- 1,600 IU vitamin E oil
- 2 tbsp. + 2 tsp. horsetail tops infused oil (p.20)
- 3 tbsp. grated beeswax

Skin-Calming Tea

This tea helps to soothe eczema and other itchy inflammations of the skin.

INGREDIENTS
Dried herbs:
- I oz. red clover flowers
- I oz. cleavers herb
- I oz. ground dandelion root
- I oz. dandelion leaf
- I oz. nettle leaves
- I oz. heartsease flowering tops
- I oz. skullcap tops

MAKES & KEEPS
Makes 7 oz.
Keeps I year.

METHOD
Mix together equal parts of the above herbs. Store in a large jar.

Shake or mix well before each use. Make tea (p.15), using 2 tbsp. of the mixture infused in 3 mugs of boiling water for 7 minutes.

Drink the 3 mugs over one day.

Take the tea for at least 3 months.

— *Tip* —

FOR ACNE, DRINK THIS TEA AND ALSO TAKE GARLIC AND ECHINACEA TINCTURE (PP.18–19), ½–I TSP. 3 TIMES DAILY. MOST PEOPLE WITH SKIN DISEASES ALSO NEED TO MAKE DIETARY CHANGES. DISCUSS THIS WITH YOUR HERBALIST OR HEALTHCARE PRACTITIONER.

Antifungal Ointment

Courtesy of Lynn Rawlinson

INGREDIENTS
- just under ½ cup coconut oil
- ¼ cup avocado oil

Essential oils:
- 8 drops lavender
- 8 drops neroli
- 4 drops myrrh
- 4 drops frankincense

MAKES & KEEPS
Makes ⅔ cup.
Keeps 6–12 months.

METHOD
Gently melt the coconut oil with the avocado oil in a double boiler or water bath. Put the oil to one side to start to cool. When the oil starts to solidify, whisk and add the essential oils. Pour the mixture into glass jars.

Apply generously to the affected area twice daily until clear of infection.

Cold Sore Ointment

Courtesy of Lynn Rawlinson

INGREDIENTS
- just under ½ cup coconut oil
- ¼ cup avocado oil
- 5 drops lemon balm (melissa) essential oil

MAKES & KEEPS
Makes ⅔ cup.
Keeps 6–12 months.

METHOD
Follow the method for Antifungal Ointment (above).

Apply a little to the affected area frequently.

Psoriasis Ointment

Courtesy of Lynn Rawlinson

Try a few different psoriasis treatments so that you find the best one for you.

INGREDIENTS
- just under ½ cup coconut oil
- ¼ cup avocado oil

Essential oils:
- 8 drops lavender
- 8 drops neroli
- 8 drops helichynum

- oil from 2 (400 IU) vitamin E capsules

MAKES & KEEPS
Makes ⅔ cup.
Keeps 6–12 months.

METHOD
Follow the method for Antifungal Ointment (opposite). Then add both the essential oils and the vitamin E oil as the ointment cools.

Apply ointment generously to the affected areas 1–2 times daily.

— *Tip* —

PSORIASIS USUALLY NEEDS INTERNAL TREATMENT AS WELL. SEE THE SKIN-CALMING TEA OPPOSITE (TAKE THE TEA AS WELL AS USING AN EXTERNAL TREATMENT). AN HERBALIST CAN USUALLY HELP PSORIASIS AND OTHER SKIN DISEASES WITH A TAILOR-MADE TREATMENT DESIGNED FOR YOU.

Psoriasis Cream

INGREDIENTS
- ½ cup Heal-All Marigold Cream (p.81)

Essential oils:
- 7 drops neroli
- 7 drops lavender
- 7 drops bergamot

MAKES & KEEPS
Makes ½ cup.
Keeps 6 months.

METHOD
Mix the essential oils into the cream.

Apply 2–3 times daily.

Psoriasis Lotion

If a large area of the body is affected by psoriasis, it is easiest to apply a lotion.

INGREDIENTS
- just under ½ cup pure vegetable glycerin

Essential oils:
- 50 drops/½ tsp. lavender
- 20 drops neroli
- 20 drops bergamot

- just under ½ cup lavender water (bought in a store or homemade, p.15)

MAKES & KEEPS
Makes just under ¾ cup.
Keeps up to 6 months.

METHOD
Whisk the essential oils into the glycerin, then gradually add the lavender water. Shake well before use.

Apply 2–3 times daily.

Acne Ointment

Courtesy of Lynn Rawlinson

A variation on the Cold Sore Ointment (p.118).

INGREDIENTS
- just under ½ cup coconut oil
- ¼ cup avocado oil
- 8 drops tea tree essential oil

MAKES & KEEPS
Makes ⅔ cup.
Keeps 6–12 months.

METHOD
Follow the method for Antifungal Ointment (p.118).

Apply frequently to acne.

Drawing Ointment

Courtesy of Neil Williams

Helps to draw out splinters or pus.

INGREDIENTS
- 1 oz. dried marshmallow root
- just over ⅓ cup olive oil
- 1 oz. dried slippery elm
- 1 tbsp. grated beeswax
- 30 drops lavender essential oil

MAKES & KEEPS
Makes just over ½ cup.
Keeps 1 year.

METHOD
In a double boiler, mix the marshmallow root in the olive oil. Simmer for 1 hour. Add the slippery elm and mix until smooth, then add the beeswax and let it melt in. Let it cool slightly for 5 minutes, then mix in the lavender oil before transferring to jars.

Apply generously to affected areas until the splinter or pus is out.

Fissure Salve

Courtesy of Stephen Buhner

Heals painful skin fissures (fingers, feet, or anal) that do not respond to other interventions.

INGREDIENTS
- 1 oz. Japanese knotweed root, dried and cut into tiny pieces
- 1 oz. Stephania root (a Chinese vine with strong anti-inflammatory effects), dried and cut into tiny pieces
- ¼ oz. dried thyme
- up to 2 cups olive oil, enough to cover
- ½ tsp. vitamin E oil
- 3–6 tbsp. grated beeswax

MAKES & KEEPS
Makes up to 2 cups.
Keeps at least 1 year in the refrigerator.

METHOD
Make an infused oil (p.20) by putting the herbs into a lidded ovenproof dish and adding olive oil to cover to a depth of ½ inch. Let sit overnight in the oven on its lowest setting.

Cool for an hour or so, strain, and measure, then add the vitamin E oil and slowly reheat, adding 2 tbsp. of beeswax per 1 cup of oil.

Apply frequently.

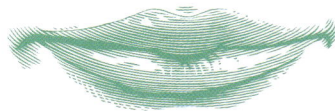

Cold Sore Lotion

Courtesy of Dedj Leibbrandt

INGREDIENTS
Tinctures (pp.18–19):
- ½ tsp./3ml myrrh tincture (this is made with 190 proof alcohol because it is a resin; see tip, p.78).
- ¾ tsp./4ml lemon balm tincture
- ½ tsp. St. John's Wort Oil (p.83)
- 3 drops lemon balm (melissa) essential oil

MAKES & KEEPS
Makes 2 tsp.
Keeps 3 years.

METHOD
Mix together in a small bottle. Dab it on frequently throughout the day, reducing as the pain of the cold sore subsides.

Antiwart Tincture

Courtesy of Karen Stephenson

INGREDIENTS
- ⅓ oz. fresh greater celandine, crushed
- 1 cup Apple Cider Vinegar (p.165)

MAKES & KEEPS
Makes about 1 cup.
Keeps 1–2 years.

METHOD
Make as for herbal vinegars (p.19).

Dab undiluted onto warts twice daily. Alternatively, use a pad soaked in the tincture and place onto the wart with a bandage. Change daily.

Wart & Verucca Zapper

Courtesy of Dedj Leibbrandt

Suitable for adults and children, the zapper is good for clusters of warts or verrucas. Be aware that persistent warts or verrucas can indicate an underlying problem or weakness.

INGREDIENTS
- 5 tsp. lemon essential oil
- 5 tsp. castor oil
- 7 tsp./35ml white cedar tincture (pp.18–19)
- 3 tsp./15ml greater celandine tincture (pp.18–19)

MAKES & KEEPS
Makes just under ½ cup.
Keeps 2–3 years.

METHOD
Mix all the ingredients together in a bottle.

Shake before each use. Cover the entire affected area twice daily. Note: It will take several weeks to take effect.

Fungal Toe Nail Cure

Courtesy of Dedj Leibbrandt

*This treatment works if used for several months—
and continued for 1 month after the nails look clear.*

INGREDIENTS
Essential oils:
Mixture 1
- 50 drops/½ tsp. cinnamon
- 1¼ tsp. lemon
- 50 drops/½ tsp. oregano

Mixture 2
- 1¼ tsp. tea tree
- 50 drops/½ tsp. thyme
- 50 drops/½ tsp. palmarosa

MAKES & KEEPS
Makes 2½ tsp. of each mixture.
Keeps 2–3 years.

METHOD
Rub mixture 1 into the nail bed once daily for
1 week. Then swap to mixture 2 and then back
to mixture 1 and so on for as long as it takes to
clear the nails.

Cancer Treatment Survival Drink

*These herbs help the body to cope with the adverse
effects of chemotherapy and radiotherapy.*

INGREDIENTS
Dried ground herbs:
- 1 oz. ginseng root
- 1 oz. milk vetch root
- 1 oz. ginger root
- 1 oz. caraway seeds

MAKES & KEEPS
Makes 4 oz.
Keeps 1 year.

METHOD
Mix the ground herbs together and jar.

Make the tea (p.15), using 2 tsp. per mug of
boiling water. Infuse for 10 minutes and drink
1 cup twice daily.

Alternatively, add 2 tsp. of the herb mixture to
your favorite smoothie.

Take it while having chemotherapy and radiation
therapy, and for a few months after to help the
immune system recover.

Radiation Therapy Healing Salve

Courtesy of Catherine Johnson

*This is particularly good for women having radiation
therapy for breast cancer. It helps the skin's integrity
and helps prevent painful reddening of the skin.*

INGREDIENTS
- just over ¾ cup Heal-All Marigold Oil (p.81)
- 2¼ tbsp. grated beeswax
- ½ tsp. blue chamomile essential oil

MAKES & KEEPS
Makes just under 1 cup. Keeps 6 months.

METHOD
Gently heat the marigold oil with the beeswax
in a double boiler or water bath until melted.
Remove from heat, let cool for 5 minutes, then
stir in the essential oil. Pour into a jar.

Gently apply to the skin over the affected area
3–4 times daily in the weeks prior to and during
radiation therapy treatment.

Caution

Wash the skin before radiation therapy. Do not use
salve for 2 hours before radiation therapy.

Blood-Cleansing Formula

This mixture, for support during cancer treatment, is based on traditional cancer treatments (including the Native American "Essiac" formula).

INGREDIENTS
Dried herbs:
- 4 oz. burdock root, finely chopped
- 2 oz. sheep sorrel leaves
- 1¾ oz. slippery elm, ground
- ⅓ oz. turkey rhubarb root

- 1 quart boiling water
- 1 tbsp. ground turmeric

MAKES & KEEPS
Makes 7¾-oz. herb mixture.
Keeps 1 year. Once made up, keeps 3 days
in the refrigerator.

METHOD
Mix all the dry ingredients together, except the
ground turmeric.

To make 1 day's dose, put ⅓ oz. of the mixture
with the water into a saucepan. Simmer, covered
with a lid, for 10 minutes. Remove from heat
and let sit overnight. The next day, bring
back to a boil and add the turmeric powder.
Remove from the heat, let sit for 15 minutes,
then strain.

Drink at least half immediately. Take the rest
over the course of the day.

Violet Salve for Tumors

Courtesy of Louise Berliner

Violet leaves are known to dissolve hardness in the body. They are traditionally used to treat lumps in the breast.

INGREDIENTS
- 2 handfuls of fresh violet leaves (and flowers)
- just over ¾ cup olive oil
- 5 tsp. grated beeswax
- 1 drop of rose essential oil
- 10 drops frankincense essential oil

MAKES & KEEPS
Makes about ¾ cup.
Keeps about 6 months.

METHOD
Pick the tiny violet leaves and flowers, and put
them into a basket to wilt for a few hours. Make
an infused oil over 5–6 weeks (p.20).

Strain off the oil and heat it gently with the
beeswax in a double boiler or water bath to melt
the wax. Then remove the mixture from the
heat, add the rose and frankincense essential
oils, and pour into jars.

Apply a little to lumps 2–3 times daily.

Caution

Consult a healthcare professional immediately if you
find a lump in your breast, or elsewhere.

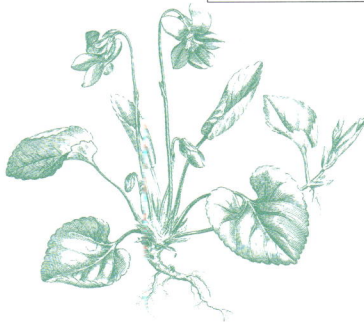

SNUFF

People have ingested herbs in ground form as a nasal snuff for millennia. It's a great strategy and can be a pleasant experience. The plant particles mop up infected reservoirs of mucus so that they can be expelled from the nose, while the good stuff in the herbs is absorbed straight into the bloodstream. Snuffs are mostly used for problems with the nose and sinuses, but they also have some generalized effects on the body.

The method for making snuffs is always the same. Measure finely ground herbs and mix together. Then rub in the essential oil (wear fine plastic gloves for hygiene). Sift 8 times, using a sifter or fine-mesh strainer, or more until the powders are blended and the essential oils mixed in.

Each recipe makes 6 tsp. of snuff and keeps at its best for 1 year. Store in a small airtight container. Take a pinch of snuff and sniff it up the nose 2–3 times daily.

All these recipes are courtesy of Melissa Ronaldson.

Uplifting Snuff

To uplift the mood.

INGREDIENTS
- 2 tsp. marshmallow root
- 2 tsp. rosemary
- 2 tsp. sweet flag
- 1 drop frankincense essential oil

Soothing Snuff

Calms sore and inflamed sinuses.

INGREDIENTS
- 2 tsp. marshmallow root
- 2 tsp. plantain
- 2 tsp. echinacea
- 1 drop chamomile essential oil

Opening & Clearing Snuff

Helps to open sinuses and clear blocked mucus.

INGREDIENTS
- 2 tsp. marshmallow root
- 2 tsp. lime flowers
- 2 tsp. elecampane

Essential oils:
- 1 drop peppermint
- 1 drop eucalyptus

Polyp Snuff

To shrink nasal polyps.

INGREDIENTS
- 2 tsp. marshmallow root
- 2 tsp. myrica
- 2 tsp. oak bark
- 1 drop frankincense essential oil

Up-All-Night-&-Still-Dancing Snuff

These herbal stimulants help to keep you going longer.

INGREDIENTS
- 22 tsp. marshmallow root
- 2 tsp. ashwaganda
- tiny pinch of black pepper
- tiny pinch of chili pepper
- 2 drops peppermint essential oil

BABIES' & CHILDREN'S RECIPES

Here, follow some safe and effective recipes for treating children and babies. All of these recipes are also suitable for adults; an adult dose is up to double the children's one.

Some of these recipes contain honey, but please note it's not recommended that you give honey to babies under 1 year old. Always consult your healthcare practitioner for any serious symptoms in young people.

Dry Bed Syrup

INGREDIENTS
- ½ oz. dried agrimony (or 1 oz. fresh)
- ½ oz. dried St. John's wort (or 1 oz. fresh)
- 1 oz. fennel seeds
- 2 cups water
- 1 (12-oz.) jar of honey

MAKES & KEEPS
Makes about 3 cups.
Keeps 1 year unopened. After opening, keep in refrigerator and use within 1 month.

METHOD
Decoct the herbs in the water (p.15). Simmer the decoction for 10 minutes, then let steep until cool. Strain. Add the honey and return to the heat to make a syrup (pp.21–22).

Give 1 tsp. at bedtime until the bed-wetting problem is resolved.

Wild Cherry Cough-Calming Syrup

INGREDIENTS
- 1 cup wild cherry root
- 2 cups water
- 1 cup cherry juice (freshly made or bought in a store)
- 2 cups white sugar

MAKES & KEEPS
Makes about 3⅓ cups.
Keeps 1 year unopened. After opening, keep in refrigerator and use within 1 month.

METHOD
Decoct the wild cherry root in the water (p.15). Simmer the decoction until reduced by about half (this usually takes 20–30 minutes). Strain and add the cherry juice and sugar. Make the syrup (pp.21–22).

Give ½–2 tsp. at night to help sleep. Also give ½–1 tsp. up to 3 times a day to calm an irritable cough (when no mucus needs to be coughed up; see box below).

Caution
The syrup suppresses coughing, which is helpful at night. However, if there is mucus that needs to be coughed up from the lungs, do not use this mixture during the day, because coughing then will rid the lungs of mucus.

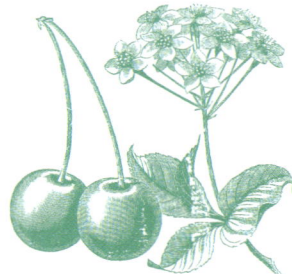

Children's Cough Honey

Courtesy of Anne McIntyre

INGREDIENTS
- 1 (12-oz.) jar of honey
- 2 tsp. holy basil leaves
- 2 tsp. thyme leaves
- 2 tsp. hyssop flowering tops

MAKES & KEEPS
Makes about 12 oz.
Keeps at least 1 year.

METHOD
Remove some of the honey so that the jar is four-fifths full. Place the herbs in a reusable tea bag (or tie them in a small piece of cheesecloth) and add to the jar. Let sit on a sunny windowsill for 3 weeks. If you want a stronger flavor, remove the bag and replace it with the same quantity of fresh herbs, then infuse for another few weeks.

Give 1 tsp. daily in a mug of hot water or ginger tea (p.15) as a preventive. Give 3–6 times daily in acute infections.

Cough Tea

This is a good alternative to cough honey (above), which is suitable for babies under 1 year of age.

INGREDIENTS
Dried herbs:
- 1 oz. holy basil leaves
- 1 oz. thyme leaves
- 1 oz. hyssop flowering tops

MAKES & KEEPS
Makes 3-oz. herb mixture.
Keeps 1 year.

METHOD
Mix the herbs together and store in a jar.

Make the tea (p.15), using 1 tsp. herb mix to 1 mug of boiling water. Put the herbs into a teapot and add boiling water. Infuse for 10 minutes.

Drink while warm, 1–3 cups daily.

Baby's First Herbal Tea

This tea both soothes and calms the digestive system and gets baby used to herbal teas.

INGREDIENTS
One or more of the following dried herbs:
- 1 oz. chamomile flowers
- 1 oz. fennel seeds
- 1 oz. lime flowers

MAKES & KEEPS
Makes 1 serving.
Keeps 1 year.

METHOD
Make a weak infusion (p.15), using 1 tsp. per mug of boiling water, brewed for 5 minutes and then strained.

Let cool and give 1–2 tsp. to baby on a teaspoon. (You can drink the rest.)

Any baby who can sip from a teaspoon is old enough for this tea. It can be served every day.

Salve for Eczema

Courtesy of Anne McIntyre

INGREDIENTS
- 1¼ cups coconut oil
- 1 handful of a mixture of marigold petals, chamomile flowers, and lavender flowers (ideally fresh), coarsely chopped

MAKES & KEEPS
Makes 1¼ cups.
Keeps 3–6 months.

METHOD
Gently heat the oil and the herbs in a double boiler or water bath for 3–4 hours. Strain and press through cheesecloth. Discard the herbs and pour the liquid into jars.

Apply generously to the affected area at night and morning, after gently washing the area with rosewater.

Meadowsweet Antidiarrhea Honey

Raw honey's antibacterial properties can help to treat diarrhea. Combined with astringent, anti-inflammatory meadowsweet, it makes a delicious and useful remedy for infants' and children's diarrhea.

INGREDIENTS
- I (I2-oz.) jar of honey
- an equal amount of strong meadowsweet tea (p.I5; make with I½ cups boiling water over I oz. dried meadowsweet/I handful of fresh)

MAKES & KEEPS
Makes 24 oz.
Keeps up to I year unopened. Once opened, keep in the refrigerator and use within I–2 months.

METHOD
Add the honey to the hot tea, stirring well until it all has dissolved. Bottle.

Give I tsp. every I–2 hours to treat an attack of diarrhea. Continue to give 2 tsp. daily for 5 days after the attack has passed.

Caution

Children can quickly become dehydrated if they have diarrhea. Replenish lost fluids with the "Lemon Sherbert" Rehydration Remedy (p.93) and seek healthcare advice.

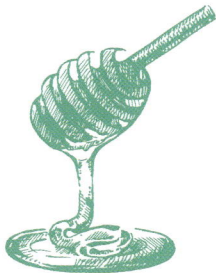

Mucus-Busting Tea

Courtesy of Anne McIntyre

INGREDIENTS
Dried herbs:
- ½ tsp. chamomile flowers
- ½ tsp. plantain leaves
- ½ tsp. elderflowers
- 2 cups boiling water

MAKES & KEEPS
Makes about I¾ cups.
Keeps 4 days in the refrigerator.

METHOD
Mix the herbs together. Pour on the boiling water and let cool. Strain.

Give 2 tbsp. in a bottle or 6 tsp. off a spoon before feeding, 3 times daily.

Teething Rub

Courtesy of Anne McIntyre

INGREDIENTS
- I tsp. dried chamomile flowers
- I mug of boiling water

MAKES & KEEPS
Makes I mug.
Keeps 4 days in the refrigerator.

METHOD
Infuse the flowers in the water (p.I5) for I hour until cool.

Strain and soak a teething ring or cloth in the cold tea.

Give to the baby to suck, or rub onto sore gums, as needed.

Sore Throat Gargle

Courtesy of Anne McIntyre

Many children love to gargle once they are old enough—which could be as young as 4 or 5, depending on the child.

INGREDIENTS
- ½ tsp. ground turmeric
- ½ tsp. sea salt
- 1 mug of warm water

MAKES & KEEPS
Makes 1 mug, enough for 1 day.
Keeps up to 3 days in the refrigerator.

METHOD
Dissolve the turmeric and salt in the water.

Gargle frequently throughout the day.

Sweet Sleep Syrup

Helps a fractious child relax into sleep.

INGREDIENTS
Dried herbs:
- 1 oz. chamomile
- ½ oz. catnip
- ½ oz. rosebuds or petals

- 2 cups rosewater
- 2 cups sugar, or 1¼ cups honey

MAKES & KEEPS
Makes about 2½ cups.
Keeps 6–12 months in the refrigerator.

METHOD
Mix all the herbs together in a saucepan and add the rosewater. Bring the mixture to a boil, then remove from the heat. Let cool, then strain. Reduce the liquid to 1¼ cups by simmering. Make a syrup with the sugar or honey (pp.21–22).

Give 1–3 tsp. in a mug of hot milk or almond milk at bedtime.

Sweet Sleep Pillow for Children

INGREDIENTS
Dried herbs:
- 1½ oz. lime flowers, finely shredded
- ¾ oz. lavender flowers
- ¾ oz. rose petals

Essential oils:
- 5 drops lavender
- 3 drops rose

YOU WILL NEED
- ABOUT 12 X 8-INCH RECTANGULAR BAG OF COTTON CLOTH/SMALL PILLOWCASE

MAKES & KEEPS
Makes 1 pillow.
Keeps effective for 6 months or more.

METHOD
Mix the herbs well in a large bowl. Sprinkle on the oils. To make the pillow, fill the bag or pillowcase with the mix and be sure it's sealed.

Place the herbal pillow beside the child's ordinary pillow.

— *Tip* —

REFRESH THE PILLOW BY ADDING A FEW DROPS OF ESSENTIAL OILS EVERY NOW AND THEN TO KEEP IT SMELLING LOVELY. AS AN ALTERNATIVE TO A PILLOW, MAKE A "TRANQUIL TEDDY" BY STUFFING A FAVORITE CUDDLY TOY WITH EITHER OF THE SLEEP PILLOW HERB MIXTURES (ABOVE AND OPPOSITE). REPLACE THE HERBAL MIXTURE AFTER 6–12 MONTHS.

Calming Herbal Baths

Courtesy of Anne McIntyre

This bath can be used daily or when a child is fussy, in pain or discomfort—or simply overenergized.

INGREDIENTS
Use 1 generous handful of any of these herbs (or mix any two or more of them):
- chamomile flowers
- lavender buds
- rose petals
- lemon balm leaves

YOU WILL NEED
- A STOCKING OR THIN SOCK

MAKES & KEEPS
Makes enough for 1 bath. If using dried herbs, you can prepare in advance; the dry mix will keep for 1 year.

METHOD
Place the herbs into a stocking or thin sock and knot it at the end to make an herbal bath bag. Tie it so that the hot water runs over it as you fill the bathtub. Fill the bathtub completely with hot water, then let it cool to a comfortable temperature. Squeeze the herbal bath bag to increase the strength of the infusion.

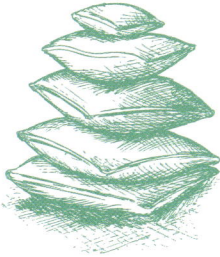

Holy Sleep Pillow

Courtesy of Anne McIntyre

Promotes sleep and pleasant dreams.

INGREDIENTS
Dried herbs:
- 1 oz. lavender flowers
- 2 oz. chamomile flowers
- 1 oz. holy basil

YOU WILL NEED
- ABOUT 12 X 8-INCH RECTANGULAR BAG OF COTTON CLOTH/SMALL PILLOWCASE

MAKES & KEEPS
Makes 1 pillow.
Keeps effective for 6 months or more.

METHOD
Make and use as for the Sweet Sleep Pillow for Children (opposite).

— *Tip* —

YOU COULD ALSO PLACE
THE HERBS LOOSE IN A BOWL
BY YOUR BEDSIDE.

Sesame & Lavender Baby Oil

Courtesy of Anne McIntyre

INGREDIENTS
- ½ cup sesame oil
- 30 drops lavender essential oil

MAKES & KEEPS
Makes ½ cup.
Keeps 6–12 months.

METHOD
Mix the ingredients together.

Apply gently over the baby's skin. Avoid contact with the eyes.

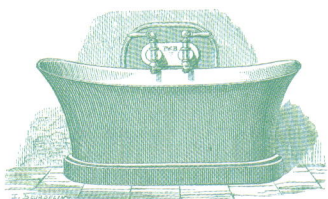

Soothing Oat Bath

A soothing alternative to bubble bath, good for any kind of itching or irritated skin. It also soothes chicken pox sores.

INGREDIENTS
- 🍃 1 cup rolled oats

YOU WILL NEED
· A SOCK

MAKES & KEEPS
Makes 1 bath.
Keeps dry for 3–6 months in the bathroom.

METHOD
Put the oats into the sock. Tie it around the hot faucet so that the water runs through the oats as it fills the bathtub. Let the water cool to a comfortable temperature.

— *Variation* —

FOR A CALM AND SOOTHING BATH, ADD SOME OF THE HERBS SUGGESTED FOR THE CALMING HERBAL BATHS (P.129) TO THE OATS.

Rash Ointment

Courtesy of Teri Evans

This will nourish your hands as well as your baby's buttocks.

INGREDIENTS
Dried herbs:
- 🍃 1 tbsp. chickweed leaves
- 🍃 1 tbsp. marshmallow root
- 🍃 1 tbsp. comfrey root or leaf
- 🍃 ½ tsp. goldenseal or baical skullcap flowering tops
- 🍃 just under 1 cup sweet almond oil
- 🍃 6 tbsp. grated beeswax

MAKES & KEEPS
Makes just under 1 cup. Keeps 2 months.

METHOD
Infuse the herbs with the almond oil (p.20). Gently cook for 2–3 hours in a double boiler. Strain, melt in the beeswax, and pour into jars.

Apply every time you change a diaper.

Vitamin Ice Pops

A good way to get healthy herbs into your child.

INGREDIENTS
- 🍃 ⅓ cup Many Berry Syrup (p.55)
- 🍃 1½ cups cooled nettle tea (p.15; make with 4 tsp. nettles infused in 1⅔ cups boiling water for 10 minutes)

YOU WILL NEED
· POPSICLE MOLDS

MAKES & KEEPS
Makes 8–10 popsicles. Eat within 3 months.

METHOD
Mix the ingredients together. Pour into popsicle molds and freeze.

Eat 1–2 daily.

Anti-Allergy Ice Pops

These can help treat hay fever and pet allergies.

INGREDIENTS
- 1½ cups nettle leaf tea
  (make as for Vitamin Ice Pops, opposite)
- ⅓ cup elderflower syrup (pp.21–22)

YOU WILL NEED
· POPSICLE MOLDS OR ICE CUBE TRAYS

MAKES & KEEPS
Makes 16–20 popsicles.
Eat within 3 months.

METHOD
Mix the ingredients well. Freeze in popsicle molds or ice cube trays.

Eat 1–3 daily.

Special Baby Wipes

Courtesy of Anna Dowding

These guarantee permanently peachy buttocks …

INGREDIENTS
- 2 tsp. best-quality Apple Cider Vinegar (p.165)
- 2 tsp. calendula tincture (pp.18–19)

Essential oils:
- 3–4 drops tea tree
- 3–4 drops lavender

- 2 tsp. vegetable oil (either coconut, jojoba, or olive)
- 2 cups of water

YOU WILL NEED
· COTTON WIPES OR COTTON BALLS

MAKES & KEEPS
Makes 100–200 wipes. Keeps 6 months or more.

METHOD
Mix all the ingredients together in a quart jar. Squash in as many wipes or cotton balls as you can to soak up the mixture. Close the jar and keep it sealed until use.

Baby Powder for Dry Buttocks

An herbal alternative to talcum powder.

INGREDIENTS
- 4 tsp. cornstarch
- 3 tbsp. baking soda
- 2 tbsp. dried chamomile flowers, ground to a fine powder
- 5 drops lavender essential oil

MAKES & KEEPS
Makes just over ½ cup.
Keeps up to 6 months in an airtight container.

METHOD
Mix all the ingredients together. Sift the mixture a couple of times. Shake well before use.

— Variation —

FOR A STRONG POWDER TO HELP PREVENT AND TREAT ATHLETE'S FOOT, ADD ESSENTIAL OILS (30 DROPS TEA TREE AND 30 DROPS LAVENDER) TO THE MIXTURE.

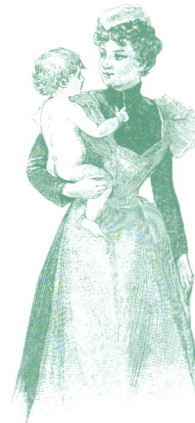

Antioxidant-Rich Sunscreen

Courtesy of Monika Ghent

This makes a moderately strong sunscreen.

Read the section on cream-making techniques (pp.20–21) before you start.

INGREDIENTS

Oil phase:
- 2 tbsp. + 2 tsp. olive oil
- ¼ cup coconut oil
- 4 tsp. shea butter
- 1½ tsp. liquid lecithin
- 1½ tsp. grated beeswax

Water phase:
- 1 tbsp. fresh aloe gel
- ¼ cup green tea infusion (p.15)
- 3 tbsp. rosewater
- 20 drops carrot seed oil

Essential oils:
- 30 drops lavender essential oil
- 5 drops rosemary
- 5 drops peppermint
- 10 drops liquid vitamin D
- 5 (400 IU) vitamin E capsules
- 10 drops Walnut Flower Remedy (p.59)
- 1 tbsp. zinc oxide

YOU WILL NEED
- A HAND BLENDER

MAKES & KEEPS
Makes 1 cup.
Keeps 1–3 months in the refrigerator.
Refrigerate between uses.

METHOD
Measure all the ingredients and have them ready to use before you begin.

Melt the oil phase ingredients in a double boiler. Put the aloe gel into a bowl and whip it into a foam with a handheld blender. Slowly drizzle the oil phase into the water phase. Blend well together for a couple of minutes.

Add the carrot seed oil, essential oils, vitamin D, vitamin E, Walnut Flower Remedy, and zinc oxide to the cream while blending.

Lice Treatment for Kids

Use this together with a good nit or lice comb.

INGREDIENTS
- 1 cup strong double decoction of quassia bark (p.15)
- 50 drops/½ tsp. tea tree essential oil (not suitable for children under 7 years)

MAKES & KEEPS
Makes about 1 cup.
Enough for a 3-day treatment.
Use immediately.
Keeps up to 4 days in the refrigerator.

METHOD
Mix the ingredients together, only adding the tea tree essential oil if treating anyone over 7 years.

Wash the hair and apply a lot of conditioner, then comb through with a nit or lice comb.

Rinse hair, towel dry, and apply the treatment all over the head from root to tip. Wrap up in a towel and let dry.

Repeat daily for 3 days, and then again after 5 days. Note: Everyone in the house needs to be treated.

— *Tip* —
YOU MIGHT WANT TO USE ½ CUP OF THIS DECOCTION TO MAKE THE NIT-DETERRING CONDITIONER (P.206).

AROMATIC WATERS

Distilling aromatic waters is a lot of fun—your kitchen will soon resemble an inventor's laboratory. You can purchase a small copper still or make your own. Aromatic waters are wonderful products to use in foods, to take as medicines and aids for well-being, and to use on the skin, whether alone or as part of other recipes. If taken as medicines, the adult dose for aromatic waters is 2 tsp. 3 times daily.

All these recipes are courtesy of Joe Nasr.

Peppermint Water

This delicious aromatic water is perfect for treating heartburn and indigestion, and as a cooling lotion if applied to the skin.

INGREDIENTS
- **5 oz. dried peppermint (or 10 oz. fresh)**
- **2½ quarts water**

MAKES & KEEPS
Makes 1¼ cups.
Keeps at least a year.

METHOD
Place the peppermint and the water together in a pressure cooker. Make following the instructions for Gripe Water (right).

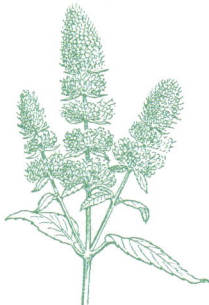

Gripe Water

Primarily to give to babies for colic, but anyone with indigestion can take this.

INGREDIENTS
Dried herbs:
- **2 oz. anise seeds**
- **2 oz. fennel seeds**
- **1 oz. dill seeds**

- **2½ quarts water**

YOU WILL NEED
- PRESSURE COOKER
- ¼-INCH SILICONE HOSE (FROM BREWER'S HARDWARE)
- POSSIBLY A HOT PLATE, DEPENDING ON THE POSITION OF YOUR STOVE

MAKES & KEEPS
Makes 1¼ cups. Keeps at least a year.

METHOD
Put the seeds and water into a pressure cooker on a counter near the sink (use a hotplate if necessary). Close the lid and remove the pressure regulator to expose the vent pipe (steam exit).

Connect the hose to the vent pipe. Pass the hose beneath the water faucet and then on and into a collecting glass bottle (10 fl. oz.).

Turn on the heat to high. When the water boils, open the faucet to let cold water flow around and cool the hose.

Simmer on low heat. To obtain a good-quality water, the distillation process should be slow with minimum heat; the distillate should not be warm to the touch but cool, ideally 95°F. Simmer until you have distilled 1¼ cups of gripe water (which in a household pressure cooker should take around 30–45 minutes).

Infants: Give 10–20 drops in water or milk up to twice daily.

Breastfeeding mothers: Take 1–1½ tsp. 3 times daily after meals.

Adults: Take 1–2 tsp. for indigestion.

Lavender Water

Aromatic water of lavender can be used on its own as a healing and calming tonic (for inside and outside the body), or added to other recipes.

INGREDIENTS
- 5 oz. dried lavender flowers (10 oz. of fresh)
- 2½ quarts water

MAKES & KEEPS
Makes 1¼ cups.
Keeps at least 1 year.

METHOD
Make in the same way as for Gripe Water (p.133).

— *Variation* —

YOU COULD SUBSTITUTE HALF THE LAVENDER FOR ROSE BUDS TO MAKE ROSE AND LAVENDER WATER.

Rosemary Water

A delicious flavoring for foods, this is also a hair tonic, a toner for the skin, and a medicine to help circulation and memory.

INGREDIENTS
- 5 oz. dried rosemary (10 oz. of fresh)
- 2½ quarts water

MAKES & KEEPS
Makes 1¼ cups.
Keeps 2 years.

METHOD
Make as for Gripe Water (p.133).

Lemon Balm Water

This lovely, lemony water uplifts the mood, helps treat headaches, and is an antiviral. It is especially good against the herpes viruses.

INGREDIENTS
- 5 oz. dried lemon balm (10 oz. of fresh)
- 2½ quarts water

MAKES & KEEPS
Makes 1¼ cups.
Keeps 6 months.

METHOD
Make as for Gripe Water (p.133).

Rose & Chamomile Water

This is a soothing skin lotion, great as a spray for hives and for sore skin, including sunburn. It can be taken internally for the stomach and the womb.

INGREDIENTS
- 4 oz. dried chamomile flowers
- 4 oz. dried aromatic rose (must be organic)
- 2½ quarts water

MAKES & KEEPS
Makes 1¼ cups.
Keeps for 6 months.

METHOD
Make as for Gripe Water (p.133)

PETS' CORNER

Animals can be treated similarly to people, although some animals should not have some herbs. Only use these recipes for the specified animals, unless advised otherwise by a qualified holistic veterinarian. These recipes are safe for home use; if in doubt, always consult a veterinarian.

For the tinctures provided by holistic veterinarian Barbara Jones, either buy the tinctures, or make your own according to the method given in the Key Preservation Techniques, pages 18–19. They all keep for 2 years or more. For all the tinctures, mix together in a bottle and use as instructed.

Valerian & Catnip Cat Toy

Cats love the smell of these herbs, particularly the valerian.

INGREDIENTS
- 1 tbsp. dried valerian root, finely chopped
- 1 tbsp. catnip

YOU WILL NEED
- MATERIAL AND A SEWING KIT TO MAKE A SMALL TOY "MOUSE"

MAKES & KEEPS
Makes 1.
Your cat will hunt the mouse down before it goes off.

METHOD
Mix the herbs well. Sew a mouse-shape small bag, leaving the tail end open. Stuff it full with the herb mixture.

Sew up tightly and add a string "tail" to the mouse.

Mange Treatment for Animals

Courtesy of Dedj Leibbrandt

This stinks, but works!

INGREDIENTS
- 3 heads garlic, coarsely chopped
- 2 handfuls of fresh elder leaves and stems, finely chopped
- 2 quarts water

MAKES & KEEPS
Makes about 1½ quarts.
Keeps 4–5 days in the refrigerator.

METHOD
Simmer the herbs in the water for 10 minutes. Remove from the heat and let sit overnight. Then strain and bottle.

Apply directly to affected areas twice daily until free of mange.

Animal Eardrops

Courtesy of Barbara Jones

INGREDIENTS
- 2 tbsp. + 2 tsp. mullein oil (p.20)
- 2 drops thyme essential oil
- 1 tsp. Heal-All Marigold Oil (p.81)
- 1 tsp. garlic infused oil (p.20; make by infusing 2 crushed garlic cloves in 2 tsp. vegetable oil, let sit for 1–2 weeks, then strain)

MAKES & KEEPS
Makes just under ¼ cup.
Keeps 6 months.

METHOD
Mix the ingredients together in a dropper bottle for easy use.

Put 2 drops into the animal's ears twice a day.

135

Scratch Pet Flea Remedy for Cats & Dogs

Courtesy of Louise Idoux

INGREDIENTS
- 4 tsp. neem oil
- 4 tsp./20ml wormwood tincture (pp.18–19)
- 3 tbsp. + 1 tsp. grapeseed oil

Essential oils:
- 2 drops lemon
- 2 drops orange
- 2 drops grapefruit
- 2 drops cedarwood
- 2 drops eucalyptus
- 2 drops citronella
- 2 drops lavender
- 2 drops sage

MAKES & KEEPS
Makes just over ⅓ cup.
Keeps 1–2 years.

METHOD
Gently melt the neem oil over low heat.
Mix all the ingredients together and bottle.

Shake before use, then rub it well into fur.
In cold weather, warm the mixture gently
before applying.

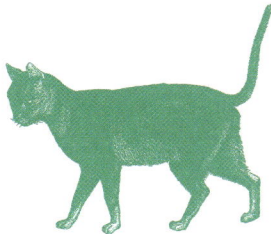

Dogs' Upset Stomach Powder

Courtesy of Barbara Jones

INGREDIENTS
- 1 oz. dried chamomile, ground
- 2 oz. dried slippery elm powder

MAKES & KEEPS
Makes 3 oz. Keeps 1 year.

METHOD
Mix together well.

Add 1 tsp. per 66 lb. weight of dog to each meal.

Alternatively, give chamomile powder on its
own, 1 tsp. with each meal.

Continue use for 1–2 days after symptoms cease.

Chronic Diarrhea Medicine for Pets

Courtesy of Barbara Jones

*Chronic diarrhea can be a symptom of something
serious; if it doesn't clear up quickly, see a veterinarian.*

INGREDIENTS
Tinctures (pp.18–19):
- 2 tbsp./30ml frankincense
- 1 tbsp./15ml echinacea
- 4 tsp./20ml goldenseal (or baical skullcap)
- 1 tbsp./15ml marigold
- 4 tsp./20ml chamomile

MAKES & KEEPS
Makes just under ½ cup.
Keeps at least 2 years.

METHOD
Mix the tinctures together in a bottle.

Give cats 3–5 drops 3 times daily.

Give dogs 1 tsp. for each 66 lb. weight of dog
3 times daily.

Pets' Mouthwash

Courtesy of Barbara Jones

For problem teeth, ulcers, and infections.

INGREDIENTS

Tinctures (pp.18–19):
- **2 tbsp./30ml marigold (made with a 190 proof alcohol)**
- **2 tbsp./30ml echinacea**
- **2 tsp./10ml goldenseal (or baical skullcap)**
- **2 tbsp./30ml chamomile**

MAKES & KEEPS
Makes just under ½ cup.
Keeps 2 years.

METHOD
Mix the tinctures together in a bottle.

Dilute 1 tsp. of the liquid in a mug of water, and flush through the pet's mouth with a syringe from side to side. Alternatively, use a sponge to apply to the gums. (Pets don't need to swallow it, although it doesn't hurt them if they do.)

Animal Eyewash

Courtesy of Barbara Jones

For sticky eyes.

INGREDIENTS

Tinctures (pp.18–19):
- **1 tsp./5ml eyebright**
- **1 tsp./5ml lemon balm**
- **1 tsp./5ml chamomile**
- **1 tsp./5ml goldenseal**

MAKES & KEEPS
Makes 4 tsp.
Use immediately.

METHOD
Bathe the eyes 2–3 times daily with ¼ tsp. in just under ¼ cup cooled boiled water. Make the eyewash fresh each time.

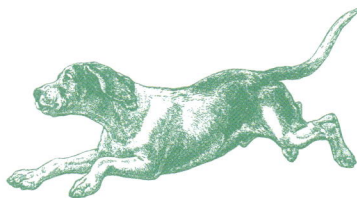

Dogs' Arthritis Medicine

Courtesy of Barbara Jones

INGREDIENTS

Tinctures (pp.18–19):
- **3 tbsp. + 1 tsp./50ml devil's claw**
- **4 tsp./20ml nettle leaf**
- **2 tbsp./30ml meadowsweet**
- **2 tsp./10ml boswelia**

MAKES & KEEPS
Makes just under ½ cup.
Keeps 2 years.

METHOD
Mix together in a bottle.

Add 1 tsp. for each 66 lb. weight of dog to food 3 times daily.

Caution

Treating cats with arthritis is more difficult because salicylates are bad for them. Consult a holistic veterinarian regarding your cat's arthritis.

Pets' Liver Tonic

Courtesy of Barbara Jones

INGREDIENTS
Tinctures (pp.18–19):
- 2 tbsp./30ml milk thistle
- 2 tbsp./30ml dandelion root
- 4 tsp./20ml schisandra berry
- 4 tsp./20ml bupleurum root

MAKES & KEEPS
Makes just under ½ cup.
Keeps 2 years.

METHOD
Mix together in a bottle.

Give cats 3–5 drops 3 times daily.

Give dogs 1 tsp. for each 66 lb weight of dog
3 times daily.

Immune Booster for Horses

Courtesy of Lesley Cunningham

INGREDIENTS
Dried herbs:
- 17 oz. rubbed nettles
- 17 oz. clivers
- 17 oz. marigold flowers
- 17 oz. dandelion leaves
- 4 oz. rose hips, chopped
- 4 oz. burdock root, chopped
- 8 oz. echinacea roots and tops, chopped

MAKES & KEEPS
A sack of mix to last around 10 weeks.
Keeps 1 year.

METHOD
Place all the ingredients in a large sack.
Mix the herbs well.

Add 3 generous handfuls to your horses'
feed daily.

Horses' Wart Remedy

Courtesy of Lesley Cunningham

An old recipe for simple warts.

INGREDIENTS
- 1 fresh dandelion root or flower stem

METHOD
Squeeze the milky white dandelion juice onto
the wart 2–3 times daily.

Continue use until the wart has gone.

For persistent warts, use together with the
Immune Booster for Horses (left).

Horses' Antifungal Hoof Paint

Courtesy of Lesley Cunningham

*Thrush in horses occurs when the frogs of the hooves
become infected.*

INGREDIENTS
- just under ½ cup of vegetable oil (walnut, grapeseed, or sunflower)

Essential oils:
- 50 drops/½ tsp. tea tree
- 50 drops/½ tsp. lavender

MAKES & KEEPS
Makes just under ½ cup, enough for about
20 applications.
Keeps 6 months.

METHOD
Mix the ingredients together in a jar.

Ask a horse expert to trim the frogs, removing
all dead tissue. Wash the hoof with strong
salt water.

Paint the whole area around the frog 2–3 times
daily, washing the hoof before each application.

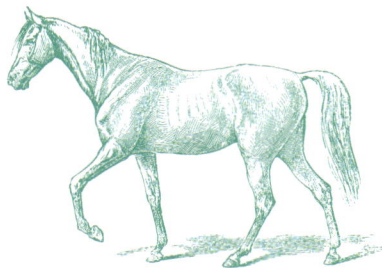

Sarcoids Cream for Horses

Courtesy of Dedj Leibbrandt

INGREDIENTS
- 6 tbsp. + 2 tsp. castor oil
- ¼ cup emulsifying wax
- ¾ cup + 5 tsp. chelidonium tea (p.15; make with 1 generous handful of fresh herb in 1 mug of boiling water, infuse for 15 minutes with the lid on, then strain)

Tinctures (pp.18–19):
- 3 tbsp. + 1 tsp./50ml bloodroot
- 3 tbsp. + 1 tsp./50ml white cedar
- Comfrey Cream for Speedy Healing (p.82)

MAKES & KEEPS
Makes almost 3¾ cups.
Keeps 1 year.

METHOD
Make the cream using the same method described for Comfrey Cream (p.82). Then mix this cream with an equal amount of Comfrey Cream.

Apply 1–2 times daily. Note: This could take a year to be effective, but it works.

Vitamin E Rich Healing Salve for Animals & People

Courtesy of Lesley Cunningham

INGREDIENTS
- just under 2 cups olive oil infused with marigold flowers (p.20)
- just under ¼ cup avocado oil
- just under ¼ cup vitamin E oil (or another just under ¼ cup avocado oil)
- ¼ cup beeswax, grated or broken into small pieces

MAKES & KEEPS
Makes about 2½ cups ointment.
Keeps at least 1 year.

METHOD
Mix the oils and make into a salve with the beeswax (see Solomon's Salves, p.117).

Apply as needed to wounds.

— *Tip* —

THIS HEALING SALVE IS GREAT FOR COWS' UDDERS THAT ARE SORE FROM MASTITIS OR OVERMILKING. IT'S ALSO HEALING FOR BREASTFEEDING MOTHERS.

— *Variation* —

FOR SKIN INFECTIONS, ADD 4 HEADS GARLIC CLOVES SEPARATED, PEELED, AND CHOPPED, AND INFUSE WITH THE MARIGOLD FLOWERS. THE GARLIC HAS A POWERFUL EXTRA ANTI-INFECTIOUS ACTION.

FOOD & DRINK

There are many wonderful things to eat and drink that can be either made with, or incorporate, interesting foraged, grown, or store-bought herbs and spices. Nature is bountiful and provides a rich variety of nourishment. In fact, wild-growing "weeds" are the true "superfoods," being often many times richer in nutrients—especially in essential minerals and vitamins—than their cultivated cousins. In recent years, there has been a resurgence of interest in foraging—gathering wild foods from nature. I hope you enjoy exploring foraging, always being careful to be certain you have gathered what you think you have before eating it. All these recipes are best eaten fresh, but most will keep 1–2 days in airtight containers in the refrigerator. Here are some ideas to whet your appetite and encourage you to start experimenting …

Probiotic Breakfast

Courtesy of Anne McIntyre

Healthful and healing breakfast for the digestive system.

INGREDIENTS

- 1 large garlic clove
- 2–4 tsp. fresh dill leaves
- 1 handful of marigold petals
- 2 tsp. fresh oregano
- 3 tsp. fresh basil
- 5 oz. carton probiotic yogurt
- 2 tbsp. aloe vera juice

SERVES & KEEPS

Serves 1.
Eat immediately.

METHOD

Add the garlic and fresh herbs to the yogurt daily for breakfast. Alternatively, take 2 tbsp. aloe vera juice with a little water or ginger tea twice daily.

— Variation —

YOU CAN USE ANY OTHER
FRESH HERBS IF YOU DON'T
HAVE THE ONES ABOVE.

Acorn Flour

Courtesy of Anna Richardson

INGREDIENTS

- 4 large handfuls of acorns (discard any with blemishes)
- several gallons of water

MAKES & KEEPS

Makes about 2 handfuls of flour.
Keeps 6–12 months, if totally dry.

METHOD

Dry the acorns for a couple of days, then remove and discard the shells. Put into a large saucepan filled with 3–4 times the amount of water to acorns. Boil for about an hour. Strain and discard the water, refill, and repeat the process two times.

Then taste an acorn; if still bitter, boil again. When they are no longer bitter, mash them and let cool a little. Strain through a strainer lined with cloth; gather the cloth and squeeze as much water out as possible.

Then spread the mush out on the cloth somewhere warm to dry. This usually takes at least 2 days. Put in a dehumidifier to speed up the process.

Grind it to flour in the coffee grinder and store in a jar. Use as ordinary flour.

Forest & Corn Goddess Cookies

Courtesy of Sharon Cohen

This recipe prepares the acorns following a different method used in the Acorn Flour recipe (opposite).

INGREDIENTS
- 1 handful of chopped acorns (or less if you have harvested fewer)
- ⅓ cup (about 5 tbsp.) melted butter
- ⅓ cup + 2 tbsp. maple tree syrup
- ½ cup hazelnut milk (at room temperature)
- ½ cup hazelnut meal (flour)
- ⅓ cup cornstarch

MAKES & KEEPS
Makes about 10–12 cookies.
Keeps 10–14 days in an airtight container.

METHOD
Preheat the oven to 350°F.

Shell the acorns and soak for a couple of days in 1¼ cups water. Change the water a few times during this period until it remains clear after a couple of hours. Boil the acorns in fresh water for 5–10 minutes, then finely chop or chop into small chunks.

Mix the chopped acorns, melted butter, and maple syrup.

Make a paste with the hazelnut milk, hazelnut meal, and cornstarch, then stir the paste into the mixture.

Place small to medium cookie-size mounds on a greased baking sheet. Bake in the oven for 12–14 minutes, then remove from the oven and let cool on the sheet.

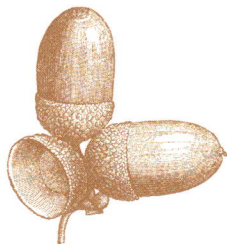

Acorn Cookies

Courtesy of Anna Richardson

INGREDIENTS
- 1 cup butter or margarine
- ¾ cup honey (or 1 cup brown sugar)
- about 3½ cups Acorn Flour (opposite)
- 1 generous cup all-purpose flour
- 1 teaspoon baking powder

MAKES & KEEPS
Makes about 30 cookies.
Keeps 10–14 days in an airtight container.

METHOD
Preheat the oven to 350°F.

Melt the butter and honey, then add the other ingredients. Stir and let cool until the dough stiffens up enough to roll into balls (golf ball size or smaller). Place the balls on a greased baking sheet and press down into flat cookie shapes. Bake in the oven for 10–15 minutes, until golden brown. Transfer to a wire rack to cool.

Caution

Acorns have been used as food by people everywhere oak trees grow. Acorns are nutritious; 1 lb. of acorns contains 2,000 calories, but they also contain high levels of tannic acid. It makes them unpalatable and toxic to the body, unless they are processed—basically washed a lot—to remove the tannins.

Plantain Seedy Oat Bars

INGREDIENTS
- 2 sticks (1 cup) unsalted butter
- 1 cup brown sugar
- ⅔ cup honey
- 4 cups rolled oats
- 2 tbsp. plantain seeds (wild-foraged)
- 2 tbsp. sunflower seeds

MAKES & KEEPS
Makes 16–24.
Keeps 10–14 days in an airtight container.

METHOD
Preheat the oven to 350°F.

Melt together the butter, sugar, and honey, stirring until the sugar is dissolved. Then add the rolled oats and seeds, and mix thoroughly. Put into an 8 x 12-inch buttered cake pan and bake for 15–20 minutes. Score when hot. Let cool, then turn out and cut.

Beech Nut Oat Bars

Beech nuts are small and difficult to handle, but they are so nutritious (rich in oils and proteins) that it's worth the effort. Gather plenty of nuts, bring them inside, and wait a day or two for the outer shells to open in the warm. Then remove the skin.

INGREDIENTS
- 2 sticks (1 cup) unsalted butter
- 1 cup brown sugar
- 200g/⅔ cup honey
- 4 cups rolled oats
- 4 tbsp. hulled beech nuts (if you can't get enough beech nuts, use 2 tbsp. beech nuts and 2 tbsp. chopped walnuts)

MAKES & KEEPS
Makes 16–24.
Keeps 10–14 days in an airtight container.

METHOD
Make as for Plantain Seedy Oat Bars (above), using beech nuts/walnuts in place of plantain/sunflower seeds.

Pharoah's Oat Bars

This recipe is inspired by sacred cakes that the ancient Egyptians offered to their gods.

INGREDIENTS
- ½ cup marshmallow root (dried or fresh), coarsely chopped/shredded
- ½ cup dates, chopped
- ¼ cup almonds, chopped
- ½ cup water
- 2 sticks (1 cup) butter
- ½ cup honey
- ⅔ cup brown sugar
- 2 tbsp. sesame seeds
- ½ cup powdered marshmallow root
- 3 cups porridge oats
- 1 cup quinoa flakes (or oats, if preferred)

MAKES & KEEPS
Makes 16–24.
Keeps 10–14 days in an airtight container.

METHOD
Let the chopped marshmallow roots, dates, and almonds soak in the water overnight.

The next day, melt the butter together with the honey and sugar. Remove from the heat and stir in the sesame seeds, powdered marshmallow root, oats, and quinoa. Add the soaked marshmallow, dates, and almonds with the water they soaked in.

Bake as for Plantain Seedy Oat Bars (left).

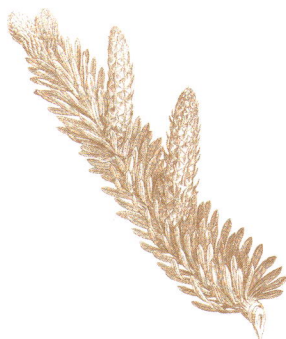

Nutty Plantain Snack

Courtesy of Karen Stephenson

INGREDIENTS

- 1 handful of plantain seeds
- 3 handfuls of pumpkin seeds
- 3 handfuls of sesame seeds
- olive oil (enough to just coat the seeds)
- sea salt, to taste

MAKES & KEEPS

Makes 7 handfuls.
Keeps 1–2 weeks in an airtight container.

METHOD

Put the seeds into a bowl, and add the olive oil and sea salt. Be sure to coat all the seeds. Either roast the seeds on a baking sheet in an oven preheated to 300°F for 10–15 minutes, or sauté in a saucepan for 5 minutes over medium heat.

Rowanberry Bitters to Stimulate Digestion

INGREDIENTS

- 4 large handfuls of fresh rowanberries
- 1 cup gin

MAKES & KEEPS

Makes about 2 cups.
Keeps 2–3 years.

METHOD

Squeeze the juice from the rowanberries using a juicer. Mix well with the gin. If you don't have a juicer, process the berries and gin in a blender and strain through a fine-mesh strainer. Then strain through cheesecloth.

Take 5–10 drops in a little water before meals to stimulate digestion, as required.

Pine Cookies

Courtesy of Karen Stephenson.

Pine needles are an excellent source of vitamin C.

INGREDIENTS

- 3 cups unbleached flour
- 1½ cups white sugar
- ½ cup pine powder (pine needles, dried and ground to a powder)
- 2 sticks (1 cup) melted butter
- 3 eggs/equivalent egg substitute
- 1 tsp. vanilla estract

MAKES & KEEPS

Makes 20–30.
Keeps 10–14 days in an airtight container.

METHOD

Preheat the oven to 325°F.

Put all the dry ingredients into a bowl. In another bowl, blend together the melted butter, eggs, and the vanilla. Combine the wet ingredients into the dry ingredients and blend well.

Roll the dough into balls about three-quarters the size of a golf ball. Place on a lightly greased baking sheet. Use a fork to flatten the cookies until they are about ¼ inch thick. Bake for 10–12 minutes.

Buckwheat Pancakes

Buckwheat contains rutin, which strengthens the blood vessels. This recipe adds in circulation-boosting herbs and is particularly good for rebuilding veins. It also tastes great.

INGREDIENTS
- I cup raw buckwheat, measured then ground
- ¼ tsp. salt
- I cup water
- 2 tsp. dried rosemary, ground
- I–2 dried horse chestnut seeds, ground—do not use more than this (optional)
- ¼ tsp. cayenne pepper or paprika
- coconut oil or butter, for frying

SERVES & KEEPS
Serves 2–4. Serve hot straight from the pan. The batter will keep uncooked in the refrigerator and can be cooked the next day.

METHOD
Make a batter by mixing the buckwheat, salt, and water and beating to a smooth batter. Let sit for ½–2 hours.

Add the rosemary, horse chestnut seeds (if using), and cayenne pepper. Beat the batter again, then heat a little oil/butter in a skillet and cook for about IO minutes on a low heat, until browned. Buckwheat pancakes cook more slowly than wheat pancakes—be patient and cook them until they look just right.

Buckwheat Blinis

Courtesy of Sucandra Devi dasi

These sweet mini-pancakes are circulation-boosters. Serve with Many Berry Syrup (p.55) for an extra boost, because blood vessels are helped by the flavonoids found in all red fruits.

INGREDIENTS
- I cup raw buckwheat, measured, then ground
- ¼ tsp. salt
- I cup water
- I tsp. ground cinnamon
- I tsp. ground ginger

SERVES & KEEPS
Serves 2–4. Serve hot straight from the pan. The batter will keep uncooked in the refrigerator and can be cooked the next day.

METHOD
Make a batter with the buckwheat, salt, water, and spices. Beat and proceed as for Buckwheat Pancakes (left).

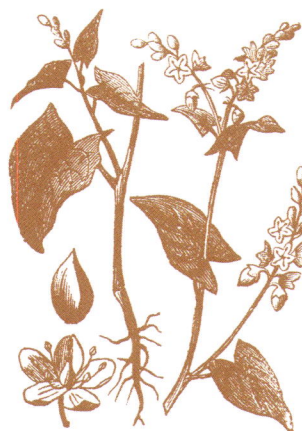

FRITTERS, PAKORAS & TEMPURA

The following fritters, pakoras, and tempura are made with a gluten-free batter made from chickpea (besan) flour.

Make a batter by mixing 1 cup of the flour with a little water, so that the paste has the texture of thick custard. Let stand for 10–30 minutes.

Chickpea (besan) flour, available in Indian grocery stores and online, is a nourishing fiber-rich food containing some healthy amino acids and minerals, and it is low in sodium and fats.

Elderflower Fritters

Courtesy of Wizz Holland

INGREDIENTS
- 6–7 heads freshly picked elderflowers
- 1 cup chickpea (besan) flour batter (see main intro recipe)
- sunflower oil, for frying
- sugar, to taste

MAKES & KEEPS
Makes 6–7 fritters.
Keeps 2 days in the refrigerator.

METHOD
Remove insects from the heads of elderflowers by placing them in a paper bag scrunched up at the top for an hour (this allows for insects to vacate) and then remove from the bag, shaking gently. Dip fresh flower heads into the batter, holding them by the stem, and deep-fry for 2–5 minutes.

When golden brown, remove from the oil and drain on paper towels. Sprinkle with sugar.

Comfrey Fritters

Packed with minerals and vitamins, these can also be made with borage leaves.

INGREDIENTS
- 1 cup chickpea (besan) flour batter (see main intro recipe)
- sweet version: ½ tsp. ground cinnamon or nutmeg; sunflower oil, for frying
- savory version: ¼ tsp. asafetida; sesame oil, for frying
- 8–10 freshly picked young comfrey leaves

MAKES & KEEPS
Makes 8–10.
Keeps 2 days in the refrigerator.

METHOD
Add either savory or sweet spices to the batter. Wipe the comfrey leaves through it, then deep-fry them for 1 minute in sunflower or sesame oil, depending on your chosen version. Drain and serve.

Pungent Pakoras

INGREDIENTS
- 1 cup chickpea (besan) flour batter (see main intro recipe)
- 1 handful of fresh wild garlic, chopped (or garlic mustard)
- 1 medium potato, chopped
- oil, for frying
- salt and black pepper, to taste

MAKES & KEEPS
Makes 8–12.
Keeps 2 days in the refrigerator.

METHOD
Mix the ingredients together. Drop a ball of the batter into hot oil and deep-fry for 1–2 minutes or until golden brown. Drain and serve hot.

Pennywort Sattvic Tempura

INGREDIENTS
- 1 cup chickpea (besan) flour batter (see main intro recipe)
- ½ tsp. wasabi powder (or ground dried horseradish root)
- 1 generous handful of pennywort leaves (or other edible greens, see p.154, Mess of Greens)
- coconut or sesame oil, for frying
- tamari or soy sauce, to taste

MAKES & KEEPS
Makes 8–12.
Keeps 2 days in the refrigerator.

METHOD
Add the wasabi or horseradish to the batter, dip the pennywort leaves in it, and fry for 1–2 minutes, until golden brown.

Drain and serve with tamari or soy sauce.

Lamb's Quarters Herbal Salt

Courtesy of Karen Stephenson

Lamb's quarters (Chenopodium album, *not to be confused with epazote), like most other wild green herbs, is rich in vitamins and minerals. This is a salt that provides for many of the body's mineral needs.*

INGREDIENTS
Dried herbs:
- 4 tbsp. dulce (or any other available seaweed)
- 2 tbsp. lamb's quarters leaves
- 2 tbsp. thyme or rosemary
- 2 tbsp. dill
- 2 tbsp. marjoram or oregano

MAKES & KEEPS
Makes 1 cup.
Keeps 3–6 months in an airtight jar.

METHOD
Gently toast the dulce using a heavy skillet or wide saucepan for a few minutes until crisp.

Grind the lamb's quarters leaves and herbs in a blender or a coffee mill while the seaweed cools. Then grind the dulce and combine with the ground herbs. Store in a shaker, and use as you would table salt.

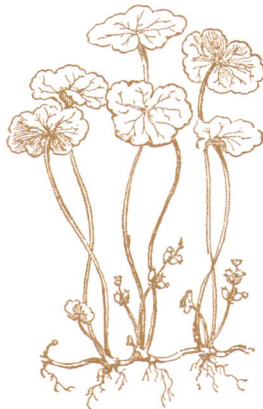

Herb Salt

INGREDIENTS

- ½ cup coarse sea salt
- 3 tbsp. fresh rosemary leaves, removed from stems
- 3 tbsp. fresh thyme leaves, removed from stems
- 3 tbsp. fresh marjoram leaves
- I cup sea salt (kosher salt is ideal)

MAKES & KEEPS

Makes 2 cups.
Keeps 6–12 months in an airtight jar.

METHOD

Put the ½ cup coarse salt and herbs into a blender and pulse to grind until well mixed (but not ground to a powder). Then add the sea salt and pulse a few times to mix well in.

Spread out to dry on a baking sheet and cover with a dish towel. Let dry for 2–3 hours. Sprinkle on raw cucumber for a tasty snack.

Wild Herb Savory Cream

INGREDIENTS

- I cup raw cashew nuts
- water, to soak
- ½ cup water
- ¼ cup mixed fresh herbs, such as thyme, sage, marjoram, wild garlic (make your own mixture from what is available)
- I tsp. miso
- juice of ½ lemon (optional)
- pinch of salt, to taste (optional)

MAKES & KEEPS

Makes I cup.
Keeps 3 days in the refrigerator.

METHOD

Soak the cashew nuts for 3–7 hours in water. Drain them and blend until smooth with the other ingredients.

Serve with crackers, or use as a spread on bread.

Rose & Cashew Cream

A wonderful alternative to dairy cream to serve with pancakes.

INGREDIENTS

- I cup raw cashew nuts
- water, to soak
- ½ cup rosewater
- I tsp. stevia powder
- ¼ tsp. cardamom powder (optional)

MAKES & KEEPS

Makes I cup.
Keeps 3 days in the refrigerator.

METHOD

Soak the cashew nuts for 3–7 hours in water. Drain and blend until smooth with the rosewater, stevia, and cardamom.

Sweet Flower Sandwiches

A lovely feast for a children's tea party.

INGREDIENTS

- 4 slices of white bread
- butter and sugar, to taste
- I handful of fresh clover flowers

MAKES & KEEPS

Makes 2 sandwiches.
Eat the same day.

METHOD

Make the sandwiches by putting the flowers on freshly buttered bread with a little sugar sprinkled on. As an alternative, try making these with primroses or violets.

Ivy-Leaved Toadflax Sandwiches

INGREDIENTS
- small handful of ivy-leaved toadflax leaves and flowers
- 4 slices rye or whole-grain bread
- butter or mayonnaise, and salt and black pepper, to taste

MAKES & KEEPS
Makes 2 sandwiches.
Eat the same day.

METHOD
Place the ivy-leaved toadflax leaves on bread freshly spread with butter or mayonnaise. Add salt and black pepper to taste. You can also make these with garlic mustard and plantain.

Pennywort Sandwiches

INGREDIENTS
- 1 handful of pennywort leaves, freshly picked and chopped
- 1 tsp. olive oil
- 1 avocado, peeled, pitted, and mashed
- 1 tsp. lime juice
- salt and black pepper, to taste
- 4 slices whole-grain bread, lightly toasted

MAKES & KEEPS
Makes 2 sandwiches.
Eat the same day.

METHOD
Mix the pennywort with the olive oil, avocado, and lime juice. Add salt and black pepper to taste. Spoon the mixture onto the bread to make a sandwich. Enjoy!

Fennel Oatcakes

Adapted from a recipe by Susun Weed

INGREDIENTS
- 2 cups rolled oats
- ½ tsp. baking powder
- ½ tsp. salt
- 1 cup oat flour
- 2 tsp. fennel seeds
- 2 tbsp. olive oil or melted organic butter
- ⅓–½ cup hot water
- ½ cup rolled oats, for rolling

MAKES & KEEPS
Makes 24–32.
Keeps 10–14 days in an airtight container.

METHOD
Grind the 2 cups of rolled oats to a fine meal in a blender or grinder—you'll get about 1½ cups of meal. Mix this with the baking powder, salt, oat flour, fennel, and oil or butter.

Add just enough hot water to form a ball of dough. Divide into 2. Sprinkle a few oats on your work surface and roll out each ball (adding more oats as needed) to about 9 inches in diameter.

Cut each circle into 6–8 wedges. Cook on a baking sheet at 350°F for 15 minutes, or in a cast-iron or other heavy skillet for 8 minutes a side.

Rosemary & Poppy Seed Oatcakes

Adapted from a recipe by Susun Weed

INGREDIENTS
- 2 cups rolled oats
- ½ tsp. baking powder
- ½ tsp. salt
- 1 cup oat flour
- 2 tsp. dried rosemary, rubbed small
- 2 tsp. poppy seeds
- 2 tbsp. olive oil or melted organic butter
- ⅓–½ cup hot water
- ½ cup rolled oats, for rolling

MAKES & KEEPS
Makes 24–32.
Keeps 10–14 days in an airtight container.

METHOD
Make as for Fennel Oatcakes (opposite), adding the rosemary and poppy seeds in place of the fennel seeds.

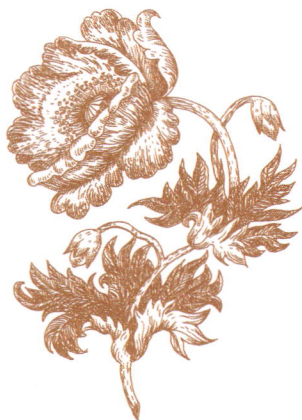

Yellow Dock Crackers

Courtesy of Karen Stephenson

INGREDIENTS
- 1 handful of yellow dock seeds, crushed
- 1 cup flour of your choice
- 1 tsp. sea salt

MAKES & KEEPS
Makes 15–30 crackers.
Keeps 10–14 days in an airtight container.

METHOD
Preheat the oven to 375°F.

Mix together the crushed yellow dock seeds, flour, and salt in a bowl. Gradually add a little water until the dough is pliable (not sticky).

Roll the dough thinly on a well-floured work surface, and cut into desired shapes.

Transfer them to a well-greased baking sheet, and bake for 10–12 minutes or until crisp.

> When you harvest yellow dock seeds for this recipe, they must be brown. Remove all leaves, stems, or anything else to be sure you have only the seeds. Store whole seeds in a paper bag. Once ground, store in an airtight jar.

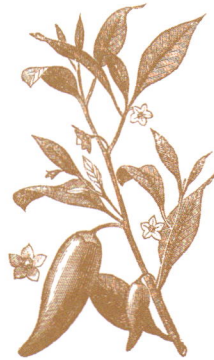

Antiflu Soup

INGREDIENTS
- 2 cups vegetable broth (see Method)
- 3–4 scallions or leeks, chopped
- 2 tbsp. coconut oil
- 2 tbsp. flour
- 1 stalk lemongrass, finely chopped
- 2 handfuls of wild greens (or spinach), chopped
- 2 cups coconut milk

SERVES & KEEPS
Serves 1–2.
Keeps 2 days in the refrigerator. Thoroughly reheat before eating.

METHOD
Make your vegetable broth by simmering a selection of vegetables in water with salt and black pepper for 1 hour. Strain and keep the liquid.

Put the scallions or leeks and coconut oil into a large saucepan and sauté on low heat for 5 minutes. Add the flour and continue to stir over the heat for 1–3 minutes, until thick.

Add the broth, lemongrass, and greens, then simmer for 15 minutes. Add the coconut milk, then simmer for an additional 5 minutes.

Sinus-Clearing Soup

Courtesy of Sue Wine

INGREDIENTS
- 4 cups water
- 1 cup sliced celery
- 1 cup thinly sliced carrots
- 2 large handfuls of fresh parsley or other green herb
- 2–3 whole green or red hot chilies
- 1 head garlic, cloves separated, peeled and crushed
- 2 tsp. miso

MAKES & KEEPS
Serves 1–2.
Keeps 2 days in the refrigerator. Thoroughly reheat before eating.

METHOD
Add all the ingredients except the garlic and miso to a large saucepan. Cover with a lid, bring to a boil, and simmer for 25 minutes. Then add the crushed garlic and cook for an additional 5 minutes, before stirring in the miso and serving.

Nettle & Wild Garlic Lentil Soup

This delicious and nourishing, mineral-rich soup is adapted from a recipe in Kitchen of Love *(2013). If you can't get the nettles and ramsons, use other wild or cultivated edible greens.*

INGREDIENTS

- 1 cup brown lentils
- 6 cups water
- 3 tbsp. olive oil
- ½ tsp. ground black pepper
- 1 tsp. asafetida, powdered
- 1 cup cubed potatoes
- 1 cup diced celery, with leaves
- 1 large handful of fresh nettle tops, chopped (wear gloves!)
- 1 large handful of freshly picked ramsons (wild garlic), chopped
- ½ roasted red pepper, cut into julienne strips
- 1 tsp. ground coriander
- 1 tsp. ground cumin
- 2 tbsp. fresh lemon juice
- 1–1½ tsp. salt, to taste
- ¼ cup each parsley and cilantro leaves, finely chopped

MAKES & KEEPS

Serves 4.
Keeps 2 days in the refrigerator. Thoroughly reheat before eating.

METHOD

Bring the water and lentils to a boil. Simmer for 15 minutes or until the lentils start to break up.

Warm the oil in another saucepan. Add the black pepper and asafetida to the potatoes and sauté over medium heat. After 2–3 minutes add the celery. Sauté for another minute, then add to the simmering lentils.

Cook for an additional 20 minutes, then add the nettles, ramsons, and all the other ingredients except the salt, parsley, and cilantro. Cook for 5–10 minutes.

Add the salt, parsley, and cilantro. Serve with bread or rice.

Nature's Bounty

These wild plants can be foraged and eaten raw or cooked (with greens, salads, stir-fries, and more).

- hawthorn leaves and blossom
- lime flower leaves
- dandelion
- garlic mustard
- wood sorrel
- sheep sorrel
- oxeye daisy leaves
- chickweed
- daisy leaves and flowers
- plantain leaves
- primrose flowers
- clover leaves and flowers
- purslane
- blackberry leaf buds
- pennywort
- violet leaves and flowers

Wild Garlic Bread

INGREDIENTS
- 1 handful of fresh wild garlic, chopped
- 2 sticks (1 cup) butter
- pinch of salt
- 1 loaf of country-style bread

MAKES & KEEPS
Makes 1 loaf.
Eat immediately.

METHOD
Preheat the oven to 350°F.

Blend the chopped wild garlic, butter, and salt together well. Make diagonal cuts along the loaf—just partway through—about 1¼ inches apart. Spread the herb butter between each of the slices.

Wrap the whole loaf in aluminum foil and place in the oven for 15–20 minutes.

Nature Smoothie

Courtesy of Shelley Harrison

This green smoothie is a mineral-rich boost that comes straight from nature.

INGREDIENTS
- 1 cucumber
- 1 avocado
- 1 handful of a mixture of 2 or more of chickweed, dandelion leaves, nettles, nasturtiums, plantain, garlic mustard, or other edible greens
- 2 cups water

SERVES & KEEPS
Serves 2–3.
Drink immediately.

METHOD
Blend everything together in a blender and serve.

Wild Garlic Pesto

Courtesy of Annie Gardner

INGREDIENTS
- ½ cup sunflower seeds (or cashew nuts or pine nuts), soaked overnight in water
- 1 tbsp. umaboshi plum seasoning
- 4–6 leaves of wild garlic (or ½ handful of garlic mustard leaves)
- 2 tbsp. olive oil
- ¼ cup water
- 1 handful of wild greens, such as chickweed, dandelion leaves, nettles, or spinach

MAKES & KEEPS
Makes about 1 cup.
Eat the same day.

METHOD
Strain and rinse the soaked seeds or nuts. Blend with the other ingredients until you reach the consistency you desire. Add more water if it is too thick.

Serve with pasta, baked sweet potatoes, or quinoa with steamed vegetables or salad. Also spread on oatcakes or bread.

Herb Pesto

INGREDIENTS
- ½ cup pine nuts, soaked overnight in water
- few sprigs fresh rosemary leaves, stems removed
- few sprigs fresh oregano
- few sprigs parsley
- 1 tsp. asafetida
- 2 tbsp. olive oil
- ¼ cup water
- 1 handful of wild greens, such as chickweed, dandelion leaves, nettles (or spinach)

MAKES & KEEPS
Makes about 1 cup.
Keeps 2 days in the refrigerator.

METHOD
Make as for Wild Garlic Pesto (above).

Calcium-Rich Herb Salad

Courtesy of Anne McIntyre

All of these nutritious herbs are rich in minerals, particularly calcium, which is vital for keeping your bones strong. The fiery arugula and nasturtium as well as the aromatic dill, cilantro, and parsley leaves will promote digestion and absorption, making sure that these vital nutrients reach your bones.

INGREDIENTS
- nasturtium flowers and leaves
- tender young plantain leaves
- young dandelion leaves
- borage flowers and leaves
- arugula
- parsley
- cilantro
- dill
- mint
- marigold flowers

KEEPS
Keeps 2 days in the refrigerator.

METHOD
Pick fresh any or all of these delicious salad herbs. Serve with a simple dressing made with olive oil and herbal vinegar.

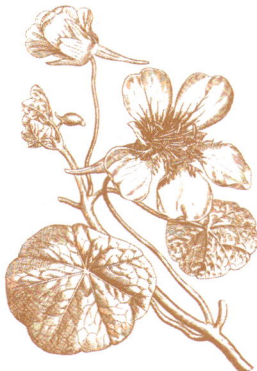

Chickweed Sag Paneer

Adapted from a recipe in Kitchen of Love *(2013).*

INGREDIENTS
- 2 tbsp. ghee or sesame oil
- 1½ tsp. cumin seeds
- 1 green chile, seeded and finely chopped
- 1 tbsp. chopped fresh ginger root
- 1 tsp. asafetida
- 1 tsp. ground coriander
- 1 tsp. ground cumin
- 1 tsp. garam masala
- 1 tsp. ground turmeric
- 3½–4 cups coarsely blended tomatoes
- 1 tsp. flour
- 10 cups chopped spinach (will shrink when cooked), lightly cooked
- 2 handfuls or 2 cups fresh chickweed, coarsely chopped and cooked
- 2 tbsp. crème fraîche or Greek yogurt
- 12 oz. paneer, cubed and fried to a light golden brown, then put into lightly salted water

SERVES & KEEPS
Serves 4–6.
Keeps 2 days in the refrigerator.

METHOD
Gently heat the ghee or oil for a few minutes and add the cumin seeds. Add the chile and ginger and reduce the heat. Add all the ground spices, stir for a few minutes, and add the tomatoes.

Mix the flour and a dash of water to a smooth paste in a small dish and add to the saucepan, stirring and cooking for a few minutes. Add the cooked spinach and chickweed, and stir for a couple of minutes.

Add the crème fraîche and mix in well. Drain the paneer from the salt water and add to the rest, simmering gently for 5 minutes.

Serve with rice and poppadoms.

Mess of Greens

To get the modern palette used to wild greens, try this recipe.

INGREDIENTS

- 6 cups dark green cabbage or kale leaves, loosely chopped
- 4–5 heads of fresh yarrow flowers, finely chopped
- 8–10 fresh nettle tops (gathered with gloves and cut up with scissors)
- 1 handful of fresh ground elder, finely chopped

SERVES & KEEPS

Serves 2–4.
Keeps 2 days in the refrigerator.

METHOD

Mix the greens and steam lightly for 4–5 minutes.

To serve, pour on a little olive oil and the herb vinegar of your choice.

Cattail Rice Recipe

Courtesy of Karen Stephenson

INGREDIENTS

- 1 tbsp. olive oil
- ½ handful of cattail shoots, peeled and chopped
- 4–6 shallots, chopped (about 1 cup)
- 2 garlic cloves, chopped
- 3 cups cooked brown rice
- 2 tbsp. tamari
- ½ tsp. cayenne pepper

SERVES & KEEPS

Serves 2–4.
Keeps 2 days in the refrigerator.

METHOD

Heat the olive oil in a large, heavy skillet. Add the cattail shoots, shallots, and garlic and sauté for 5 minutes. Add the remaining ingredients and cook until the rice is hot. Stir frequently to prevent it from sticking.

Gobō—Burdock Roots Japanese-style

Courtesy of Louise Berliner

INGREDIENTS

- 1 tbsp. sesame oil
- 1–2 burdock roots, cut into matchstick-size pieces
- 2 medium carrots, cut into matchstick-size pieces
- 1–2 tbsp. rice wine or Gorse Wine (p.177) (optional)
- 2 tsp. tamari
- 1-inch piece fresh ginger root, grated
- 1–2 tsp. toasted sesame seeds

SERVES & KEEPS

Serves 2.
Keeps 2 days in the refrigerator.

METHOD

Heat the oil and sauté the burdock root until covered in oil. Layer the carrots on the top, and add a little water (and/or wine if using) to just cover the burdock.

Cover with a lid and cook over medium-low heat for 10–15 minutes. Add the tamari and simmer. Once the liquid has almost simmered away, add the ginger, toss, and add the toasted sesame seeds.

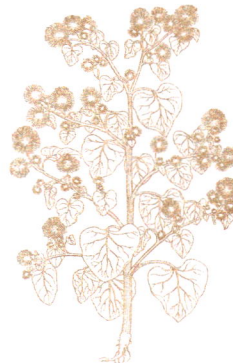

Buttered Burdock Stems

INGREDIENTS
- 2 handfuls of burdock stems
- butter and herb salt and black pepper, to taste

SERVES & KEEPS
Serves 4–6.
Keeps 2 days in the refrigerator.

METHOD
Choose young plants and cut stems close to the ground. Cut the leaves away. Wearing gloves (they will stain your hands), peel away the grayish covering skin on the stems to reveal bright green inner stems.

Steam the burdock in a steamer for 6–10 minutes, until tender. Serve hot with butter, herb salt, and black pepper. Alternatively, eat the stems cold, chopped up and drizzled with an herbal vinegar (pp.163–65).

Roasted Reed Rhizomes

Courtesy of Karen Stephenson

A delicious foraged meal.

INGREDIENTS
- 12 reed (Phragmites) rhizomes (at least 6 inches in length)
- 2–3 tbsp. olive oil
- sea salt and black pepper (or nutmeg if preferred), to taste

SERVES & KEEPS
Serves 4.
Keeps 2 days in the refrigerator.

METHOD
After washing the Phragmites rhizomes, coat them with olive oil and spices.

Place on a baking sheet. Bake at 350°F for 25 minutes.

Angelica Supreme

This is a delicious Icelandic speciality. Angelica roots and stems are also good to eat raw—try them with a dip.

INGREDIENTS
- 1 handful of young angelica stems, freshly picked
- 2 tbsp. butter (plus a little extra)
- 2 tbsp. all-purpose flour
- 2¼ cups milk
- salt and black pepper, to taste

SERVES & KEEPS
Serves 1–2.
Keeps 2 days in the refrigerator.

METHOD
Prepare the stems as for Buttered Burdock Stems (left), either steaming or boiling until soft. Put a pat of butter on them and place in a casserole dish.

Make a white sauce by gently melting the butter and stirring in the flour, and cooking for 1–2 minutes. Gradually add the milk, a little at a time, stirring all the time and cooking for about 8 minutes to make a thick sauce. Add salt and black pepper.

Pour the sauce over the angelica stems. Bake for 10–15 minutes in a warm oven.

Hot Oil

This versatile oil can be used in cooking to spice up dishes, or as a lotion for aching muscles.

INGREDIENTS
- 1 cup olive oil
- ¼ cup cayenne pepper
- ¼ cup ground ginger

MAKES & KEEPS
Makes 1 cup. Keeps 1 year.

METHOD
Make as for an infused oil (p.20).

Wild Greens

INGREDIENTS

- 1 generous handful of fresh kale, spinach, or other greens, shredded
- 1 handful of chickweed
- 4–5 fresh borage leaves (if available)
- 1 small handful of fresh violet leaves and flowers
- pat of butter or splash of olive oil
- pinch of nutmeg and herb salt (to taste)

SERVES & KEEPS

Serves 2–4.
Eat same day.

METHOD

In a steamer, lightly steam the kale for 3 minutes. Add the chickweed, borage, and violet leaves and cook for another 2 minutes.

Serve with a pat of butter and a little herb salt.

Wild Toothwort Sauce

Courtesy of Karen Stephenson

Toothwort is milder and a tiny bit sweeter than horseradish. Try this dip with fries or with Yellow Dock Crackers (p.149).

INGREDIENTS

- 3 tbsp. toothwort root, finely chopped
- 2 tbsp. sour cream
- 3 tbsp. mayonnaise or egg-free substitute
- cracked pepper, to taste
- ¼ tsp. cayenne pepper (or to taste)

MAKES & KEEPS

Makes ½ cup.
Keeps up to 4 weeks in the refrigerator.

METHOD

Simply combine all the ingredients in a mixing bowl and blend well.

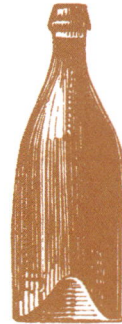

Hot Cayenne Tincture for Chili Hot Chocolate & More

Use 5–20 drops of this fiery tincture to spice up a drink or a dish.

This is known as "capsicum forte" because it is seriously strong. Cayenne is a good addition to many medicines, because it stimulates the circulation and helps with absorption of herbs.

INGREDIENTS

- ¾ cup cayenne pepper
- 2 cups organic vodka

MAKES & KEEPS

Makes 2 cups.
Keeps indefinitely.

METHOD

Make as for tinctures (pp.18–19) and store in a dropper bottle. Be careful: Wear gloves when straining and do not get this tincture in your eyes.

Add around 10 drops to a mug of hot chocolate, to taste.

Experiment with how much to add to cooking, according to taste.

As a warming and stimulating medicine, take 5–20 drops in a mug of warm water.

Horseradish Sauce

This makes a traditional and strong sauce.

INGREDIENTS
- **3 tbsp. fresh grated horseradish root**
- **2 tbsp. sour cream**
- **3 tbsp. mayonnaise or egg-free substitute**
- **Cracked pepper, to taste**

MAKES & KEEPS
Makes about ½ cup.
Keeps up to 4 weeks in the refrigerator.

METHOD
Combine all the ingredients in a mixing bowl and blend well.

Red Clover Syrup

Full of calcium and other minerals, this absolutely delicious syrup is gorgeous with pancakes—and also is medicinal.

INGREDIENTS
- **1¼ cups water**
- **3 cups white sugar**
- **2 handfuls of fresh red clover flowers**

MAKES & KEEPS
Makes about 3¾ cups.
Keeps up to a year until opened, then up to 1 month in the refrigerator.

METHOD
Make the syrup (pp.21–22) by boiling the water and sugar briskly for 3 minutes. Then pour the plain syrup over the flowers in a bowl and let sit for 1–2 hours until cool. Strain and bottle.

Hawthorn Flower Syrup

Courtesy of Lucy Wells

Hawthorn flowers make a tasty syrup that preserves their heart-strengthening and uplifting qualities.

INGREDIENTS
- **1¼ cups water**
- **3 cups white sugar**
- **7 tbsp. rosewater**
- **¼ cup lemon juice**
- **2 good handfuls of freshly picked hawthorn flowers, twigs removed**

MAKES & KEEPS
Makes about 3¾ cups.
Keeps up to a year until opened, then up to 1 month in the refrigerator.

METHOD
Make the syrup (pp.21–22) by boiling the water and sugar briskly for 3 minutes. Mix the rosewater and lemon juice with the syrup. Then pour over the flowers in a bowl and let rest for 1–2 hours, until cool. Strain and bottle.

Forsythia Syrup

Courtesy of Karen Stephenson

Capture the joyous yellow of forsythia with this tasty syrup.

INGREDIENTS
- **3 cups water**
- **3 cups white sugar**
- **3 handfuls of fresh forsythia flowers, rinsed**

MAKES & KEEPS
Makes about 4 cups.
Keeps 3 months in the refrigerator.

METHOD
Make the syrup (pp.21–22) by boiling the water and sugar briskly for 3 minutes. Then pour the plain syrup over the flowers in a bowl and let sit for 1–2 hours until cool. Strain and bottle.

Queen Anne's Lace Jelly

Courtesy of Karen Stephenson

INGREDIENTS

- 2 handfuls of fresh Queen Anne's lace flowers
- 4 cups boiling water
- ¼ cup lemon juice
- 1 (2-oz.) package powdered pectin
- 3½ cups + 2 tbsp. white sugar

MAKES & KEEPS

Makes about 5 (10-oz.) jars.
Best to use within 1 year. For long-term storage, process in a hot water bath, following USDA recommendations for home canning.

METHOD

Steep the flowers in the water, covered, for 30 minutes, then strain. Measure 3 cups of the liquid into a large, stainless steel saucepan. Add the lemon juice and pectin. Bring to a rolling boil, stirring constantly. Add the sugar and continue to stir.

Cook and stir until the mixture comes to a rolling boil, then boil for another 1 minute. Remove from the heat.

Skim the scum off the top and discard. Pour into sterilized jars leaving ¼ inch free at the top for a "head space." Sterilize the loosely sealed jars in a hot water bath for 5 minutes.

Spiced Hawthorn & Rowanberry Jelly

Full of vitamin C, this is delicious on oatcakes or with savory dishes.

INGREDIENTS

- 2 lb. rowanberries, spigs removed
- 2 lb. hawthorn berries, spigs removed
- 2 lb. crab apples, halved
- 2 cinnamon sticks, broken up
- 6 cloves (optional)
- water and sugar (variable quantity)

MAKES & KEEPS

Makes up to 11 lb. of jelly.
Keeps 1–2 years. For long-term storage, process in a hot water bath, following USDA recommendations for home canning.

METHOD

Put the berries and apples together with the spices in a large stainless steel saucepan, adding enough water to cover. Bring to a boil, then simmer for 30 minutes. Mash and let cool for 1–2 hours.

Pour into a double layer of cheesecloth (or jelly bag) and let sit overnight to drip through slowly. In the morning, measure the liquid, then pour into a saucepan and bring to a boil. For every 2½ cups of liquid, add 2 cups of sugar, then bring to the boil again. Boil for 1 minute, then remove from the heat. Prepare and jar your jelly as for Queen Anne's Lace Jelly (left).

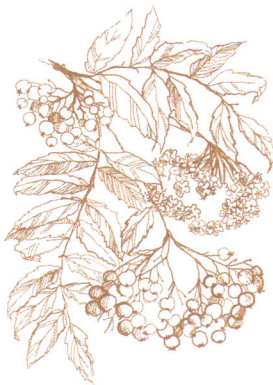

Spicy Elder & Bilberry Rob

A rob is a fruit syrup that is boiled down to a thick paste, sometimes made without added sugar when using naturally sugar-rich fruit. Add hot water to make it into a wonderful hot drink—not only tasty but also an immune-boosting tonic and a cold and flu remedy.

INGREDIENTS
- several heads/4 cups fresh elderberries, stripped from the stems
- 1 cup bilberries or blueberries
- 1 cup water
- 2 cinnamon sticks
- 8 cloves
- ½ nutmeg, grated
- up to 1 cup white sugar (variable)

MAKES & KEEPS
Makes about 1 cup.
Keeps up to a year before opening if made well and stored in sterilized jars. Keep in the refrigerator and use each jar within 3–4 weeks once opened.

METHOD
Bring the berries to a boil with the water, then cover with a lid and simmer for 2 hours. Mash the mixture well, then press out thoroughly through cheesecloth. (Wear gloves if you don't want purple hands.) Add the spices and 1 cup white sugar for every 2 cups of juice. Return to the heat and simmer for 40 minutes. Strain through a strainer and pour into sterilized jars.

Take a generous spoonful daily or more often to protect against colds and flu.

Radharani's Favorite Ice Cream

A simple and delicious ice cream, fit for a goddess.

INGREDIENTS
- 1 cup heavy cream
- ½ cup Elderflower Syrup (p.162, or Hawthorn Flower Syrup or Red Clover Syrup, p.157)
- 1 cup condensed milk

MAKES & KEEPS
Makes 8–12 servings.
Keeps 1 month in the freezer.

METHOD
Beat the cream for 1–2 minutes, then mix with the elderflower syrup and condensed milk.

Put into a freezeproof container then freeze. It should be ready in 2–3 hours.

After-Dinner Mouth Freshener

Similar recipes are known in India as Mukhwas ("mouth freshener").

INGREDIENTS
Dried seeds:
- 2 tsp. anise
- 2 tsp. fennel
- 2 tsp. lovage
- 2 drops peppermint essential oil

MAKES & KEEPS
Makes 6 tbsp.
Keeps 6–12 months.

METHOD
Mix the seeds together and sprinkle with peppermint oil. Shake well and store in an airtight container.

Chew a sprinkle of seeds after a meal.

Sweet Pickled Purslane Stems

Courtesy of Karen Stephenson

INGREDIENTS

- ¼ cup fine sea salt
- 4 cups ice-cold water
- 3–4 handfuls of fresh purslane stems, washed and removed from leaves (the leaves can be eaten)
- 2 large onions
- 1½ cups Apple Cider Vinegar (p.165)
- 2 cups white sugar
- 1 tbsp. mustard seeds
- ½ tsp. turmeric powder
- 1 cup water

MAKES & KEEPS

Makes 3 (½–quart) jars.
Keeps in the refrigerator for 6 months.

METHOD

Mix the salt and iced water, and put the purslane and onions into it for 1–2 hours in the refrigerator.

Heat the remaining ingredients to boiling point, stirring occasionally. Add the drained purslane and onions, and boil for 5 minutes. Let cool for 30–60 minutes.

Spoon the onions and purslane into canning jars using a slotted spoon, then pour in the juice to fill each jar.

Pickled Ginger

Pickle lovers will eat these on their own, or with sushi—or with any meal!

INGREDIENTS

- 2 cups thinly sliced fresh ginger root
- 8½ cups boiling water
- 2 cups rice or white distilled vinegar
- ¾ cup superfine or granulated sugar
- 1 tbsp. salt
- 1 nutmeg, grated (optional)

MAKES & KEEPS

Makes almost 3¾ cups.
Keeps in the refrigerator for up to 6 months.

METHOD

Drop the ginger into the boiling water and let boil for 3 minutes. Drain well and place in a sterilized 1-quart jar (p.17).

Heat together the vinegar, sugar, salt, and nutmeg, if using, and boil for 5 minutes. Pour over the ginger slices, put the lid on, and let cool overnight before refrigerating. This is ready to eat the next day.

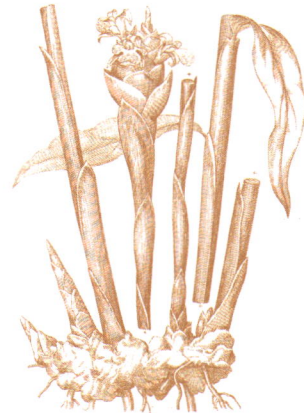

Marshmallow Candies

Nothing like the modern version, full of glucose and gelatin, these rich candies can also calm and heal the stomach and the lungs.

INGREDIENTS
- about 2½ tbsp. honey
- 1 oz. dried marshmallow root, powdered

MAKES & KEEPS
Makes 14–20 candies.
Keeps 1–2 months in an airtight container.

METHOD
Warm the honey and mix in the root to make a stiff paste. Roll into balls and let cool.

— *Tip* —
IF YOU PUT A LITTLE ALMOND OIL ON YOUR FINGERS BEFORE ROLLING THE CANDIES, IT STOPS THEM FROM STICKING.

Elecampane Candies

These delicious sweets also help the digestion and the lungs.

INGREDIENTS
- 2½ tbsp. honey
- 1 oz. dried elecampane root, powdered

MAKES & KEEPS
Makes 14–20 candies.
Keeps 1–2 months in an airtight container.

METHOD
Make and store in the same way as marshmallow candies (above).

Pure Licorice

For licorice lovers, a method of making pure solid licorice.

INGREDIENTS
- 18 oz. dried licorice, coarsely chopped
- 21 cups water

MAKES & KEEPS
Makes about 7 oz. solid licorice extract.
Keeps indefinitely.

METHOD
Decoct the licorice in the water (p.15), simmering covered for 30 minutes. Strain well through cheesecloth.

Heat the decocted liquid in a double boiler or water bath, letting the water evaporate off until the licorice extract becomes more concentrated. After 1½ hours, you will be left with an almost solid, sticky black goo.

Put the mixture into molds or flat on a greased and lined baking sheet. Let sit to continue drying out for about 2 weeks (though in warm climates, or if you use a dehumidifier, this can take only 5 days). Once your licorice has dried (it will become solid), cut into pieces. You can eat it as candies or dissolve in water to use in other recipes.

Caution
For some, eating excessive amounts of licorice can raise the blood pressure and cause edema (water retention), so don't regularly eat more than 1–2 small pieces daily. Diabetics should be aware that licorice is high in sugar.

Crystallized Ginger

INGREDIENTS

- 4½ cups fresh sliced ginger root
- 5 cups water
- 2 cups white sugar

MAKES & KEEPS

Makes almost 1½ lb.
Keeps 2 weeks in an airtight container.

METHOD

Cook the ginger in the water for 20 minutes until soft. Drain and reserve ¼ cup of the cooking water.

Mix together the ginger, reserved cooking water, and sugar. Simmer, stirring, for about 20 minutes until most of the water has evaporated and the syrup is beginning to crystallize. Then spread the ginger pieces out on a rack to cool.

— Variation —

YOU CAN MAKE A SIMILAR MIX
USING MARSHMALLOW, ANGELICA,
ELECAMPANE, DANDELION, AND
OTHER ROOTS.

Elderflower Syrup

This delicious syrup (called a cordial in other countries) is wonderful mixed with sparkling water.

INGREDIENTS

- 2½ cups white sugar
- 3 cups boiling water
- 20 heads fresh elderflowers, insects removed as in Elderflower Fritters (p.145)
- 4 lemons, the zest grated and the fruit sliced
- 1 oz. citric acid powder (a preservative; optional)

MAKES & KEEPS

Makes about 4 cups.
Keeps in refrigerator; once opened, use within 3 months.

METHOD

Make a syrup with the sugar and water in a large saucepan (pp.21–22). Add the elderflowers, lemon zest and pieces, and the citric acid, if using, and stir.

Let steep with the lid on for 2 days in a cool place, then strain through cheesecloth and store in sterilized jars.

Use as you would any syrup. Or pour indiluted over ice cream for a delicious treat.

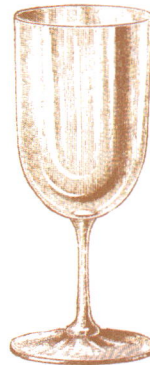

HERBAL VINEGARS

In herbal vinegars, the healing and nutritional properties of vinegar are united with the aromatic and health-protective effects of mineral-rich green herbs. They can be taken as medicines or used in a variety of ways with food: poured over beans or grains, in salad dressings, or to season stir-fries and soups.

The following herbal vinegars are made in the same way, with the herbs being infused in the vinegar for several weeks (p.19).

Quantities are provided below as a guide, but often the amount you use will depend upon how much of a particular herb you can find, grow, or pick—and on the size of jar you are trying to fill.

For internal use, always make with Apple Cider Vinegar (p.165); for external use (hair and skin washes) or cleaning products, you can use white distilled vinegar if you prefer. For use in laundry rinses, make with 1–2 tsp. per 1 cup white distilled vinegar.

If adding to food, try the vinegars in combination with cold-pressed olive oil to make a healthy salad dressing. As a medicine, take 1–2 tsp. with a little water, three times a day.

Vinegars will keep for at least 2 years in the refrigerator.

Ramsons Vinegar

Courtesy of Rachel Corby

This delicious garlicky addition to salad dressings and rice is antioxidant and antiseptic, so also makes for a powerful immune boost.

INGREDIENTS
- 1 cup wild garlic leaves, finely chopped
- 1½ cups Apple Cider Vinegar (p.165)

MAKES
Makes 1½ cups.

METHOD
See introduction and key techniques section (left and p.19).

Goldenrod Vinegar

Courtesy of Karen Stephenson

Delicious with pasta and cabbage, this vinegar will improve your mineral balance, help prevent kidney stones, eliminate flatulence, and improve immune functioning.

INGREDIENTS
- 1 cup fresh goldenrod leaves and flowers
- 2 cups Apple Cider Vinegar (p.165)

MAKES
Makes almost 2 cups.

METHOD
See introduction and key techniques section (left and p.19).

Cleavers Vinegar

Courtesy of Sensory Solutions

Helps to support the lymphatic system to clear toxins and to cool "hot" skin conditions, such as dermatitis or eczema. It is also used as a diuretic to help with edema, and to support cancer treatments. Try with wild salad or greens, or as a drink.

INGREDIENTS
- **I cup fresh cleavers herb**
- **2 cups Apple Cider Vinegar (p.165)**

MAKES
Makes just under 2 cups.

METHOD
See introduction and key techniques section (p.163 and p.19).

Balsamic Vinegar

Courtesy of Karen Stephenson

INGREDIENTS
- **I cup white pine needles**
- **2 cups Apple Cider Vinegar (p.165)**

MAKES
Makes just under 2 cups.

METHOD
See introduction and key techniques section (p.163 and p.19). Let the vinegar infuse for 6 weeks.

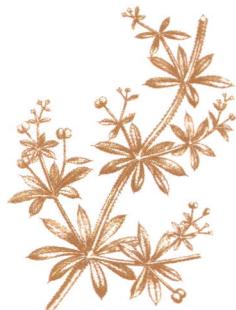

Lemon Balm Vinegar

Courtesy of Sensory Solutions

Lemon balm vinegar tastes delicious and goes well with any savory dish or salad. Lemon balm has been known as "heart's delight," because of its use to dispel melancholy.

INGREDIENTS
- **I cup fresh lemon balm flowering tops**
- **2 cups Apple Cider Vinegar (p.165)**

MAKES
Makes just under 2 cups.

METHOD
See introduction and key techniques section (p.163 and p.19).

Oregano Vinegar

Courtesy of Sensory Solutions

Perfect for an Italian-style salad dressing, you can also use it diluted as a gargle for inflamed tonsils or for a head cold. Oregano vinegar is perfect to rebalance digestion flora.

INGREDIENTS
- **I cup fresh oregano flowering tops**
- **2 cups Apple Cider Vinegar (p.165)**

MAKES
Makes just under 2 cups.

METHOD
See introduction and key techniques section (p.163 and p.19).

Rose Vinegar

Makes a beautiful pink vinegar with a subtle rose aroma. Good in salad dressings and useful for the skin and hair. Take as medicine as a liver tonic and an uplifting herb for grieving.

INGREDIENTS
- 1 cup fresh fragrant rosebuds or petals
- 2 cups Apple Cider Vinegar (p.165)

MAKES
Makes just under 2 cups.

METHOD
See introduction and key techniques section (p.163 and p.19).

Fire Cider

Courtesy of Karen Stephenson

This spicy hot vinegar goes well with tomato juice or as a straight shot to fight off colds. You can also use it externally as a muscle rub.

INGREDIENTS
- 1¼ cups Apple Cider Vinegar (p.165)
- 1 fresh horseradish root, grated (making about 1 cup)
- 5 garlic cloves, chopped
- 1–2 onions, chopped
- 3–4-inch piece fresh ginger root, grated
- 1 tsp. fresh grated cayenne pepper (or ½ tsp. dried powdered cayenne if you can't get fresh)

MAKES
Makes about 4 cups.

METHOD
See introduction and key techniques section for method (p.163 and p.19), steeping for 8 weeks.

Apple Cider Vinegar

Vinegar is made by using a "mother"—a culture of bacteria that forms during the fermentation process. This mother feeds off the sugars in the fruit, converting them to vinegar.

INGREDIENTS
- 5 apples, quartered
- water, enough to cover

MAKES & KEEPS
Makes a variable amount.
Each batch keeps for 2 years or more.

METHOD
Let the apples brown in the air, then put them into a large saucepan—the pan should be large enough so that they don't come up to the very top—and cover them with water.

Cover the pan with a thin cloth and let sit in a warm, dark place. Check it every day, stirring to aerate the mixture and skimming off any froth that comes to the top. After a few days, it will start developing a thicker layer on top—this is the vinegar mother beginning to grow. Stop stirring at this point. The liquid will become clearer as the vinegar flavor develops.

After a month, start tasting the mixture by carefully taking a little liquid out with a clean spoon. When you like the tartness, strain the liquid through cheesecloth and put into sterilized jars or bottles for use. It is normal for a sediment to form in the standing jars.

Be aware: The first time you brew this, it will take a couple of months to get the taste right; however, subsequent batches will be quicker. Once you have your vinegar mother established, you can simply add more water and apple scraps to the jar and let ferment.

To clean the jar, carefully remove the mother before lightly rinsing the jar with water. Do not use soap.

Vinegar mothers have been known to last for generations.

Lemon Barley Water

A thirst-quenching drink that is also soothing for the kidneys and bladder. Drink it regularly if you are prone to cystitis.

INGREDIENTS
- ½ cup pearl barley
- zest and juice of 1 lemon
- 2 cups boiling water
- 2–3 tbsp. honey or sugar

MAKES & KEEPS
Makes 2 cups.
Drink in 1–2 days. Keep in the refrigerator.

METHOD
Rinse the barley, then cover it and the lemon zest with boiling water. Simmer for 10 minutes, replacing the lost water. Strain the water off and set the barley aside (it is delicious to eat).

Add the lemon juice and honey or sugar to taste.

Easy Cherry Syrup

Delicious on pancakes

INGREDIENTS
- 2 cups pure cherry juice (a carton is fine)
- 2 cups white sugar

MAKES & KEEPS
Makes about 3 cups.
Keeps 3 months in the refrigerator.

METHOD
Boil the ingredients for 15 minutes to make a thickish syrup (pp.21–22).

Chai Tea with Redbush

Adapted from a recipe in Kitchen of Love *(2013).*

A delicious, caffeine-free chai.

INGREDIENTS
- 1 cup water
- 2 redbush tea bags
- 3 cloves
- 1 star anise
- 1 cinnamon stick
- ½ tsp. dried ground cinnamon
- ¼ tsp. ground black pepper
- 1½ cups milk or dairy alternative
- sweetener, to taste

SERVES & KEEPS
Serves 2.
Drink immediately.

METHOD
Bring the water, tea bags, and spices to a boil. Add the milk and sweetener and simmer for 5–10 minutes. Strain and serve.

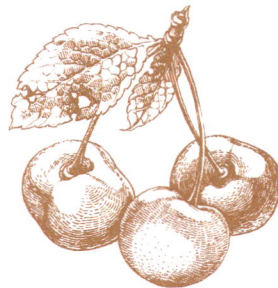

Saffron & Rose Tea

A lovely tea, rich in antioxidants.

INGREDIENTS
- few strands dried saffron
- 1 dried rosebud
- 1 mug boiling water

MAKES & KEEPS
Makes 1 mug.
Drink immediately.

METHOD
Infuse (p.15) for 5–10 minutes. Strain
and serve.

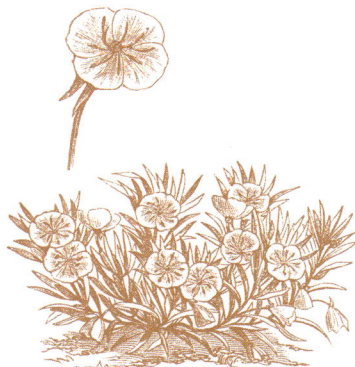

Rosemary & Lovage Lemonade

INGREDIENTS
- 4 cups water
- ¼ cup honey
- zest of 1 lemon
- juice of 3 lemons
- 3 sprigs fresh rosemary, stripped
- 3 sprigs fresh lovage, chopped
- borage, primrose, or nasturtium flowers, to garnish

MAKES & KEEPS
Makes 4 cups.
Keeps in the refrigerator up to 3 days.

METHOD
Boil the water and dissolve the honey in it.
Add the zest and let cool.

Add the lemon juice and herbs and mix well.

Chill for 2 hours, then serve, garnished with
the flowers.

Primrose & Violet Lemonade

INGREDIENTS
- 4 cups water
- ¼ cup honey
- zest of 1 lemon
- juice of 3 lemons
- 1 handful of fresh primrose flowers
- ½ handful of fresh violet leaves and flowers
- primrose flowers, to garnish

MAKES & KEEPS
Makes 4 cups.
Keeps in the refrigerator up to 3 days.

METHOD
Make in the same way as Rosemary & Lovage
Lemonade (left), but replacing the herbs with
the flowers.

Dandelion & Burdock

INGREDIENTS

For the plant "mother":
- about 6-inch piece fresh dandelion root, grated
- about 6-inch piece fresh burdock root, grated
- ½ star anise

For the pop:
- 21 cups boiling water
- 1½–2½ cups white sugar
- 2 oz. burdock root, fresh or dry
- 2 oz. dandelion root, fresh or dry
- juice of 1 lemon or lime

MAKES & KEEPS

Makes just over 5 quarts.
Keeps at least 2–3 months.

METHOD

To make the plant "mother," make as for Ginger Pop (right), using fresh grated dandelion and burdock roots instead of ginger, and adding ½ star anise to the starter (this gives the drink its hint of licorice flavor).

Add about 1 tbsp. of each root every day or two to your starter mix. Usually it's ready to use in about a week.

To make the pop, first decoct each of the roots together with 4 cups water for 30 minutes (p.15). Add another 15 cups boiling water and the sugar (add more if you want it sweeter). Dissolve, add lemon (or lime) juice, and let cool. Add your strained starter when it has cooled to 80°F and proceed as for Ginger Pop (right).

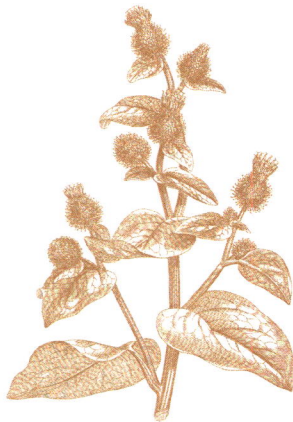

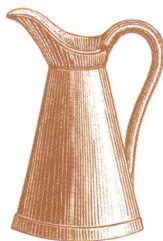

Ginger Pop

Making ginger pop is similar to making a home-brewed vinegar. The first time you make it, it takes longer to get the ginger beer "mother" started, but later batches are quicker.

INGREDIENTS

For the ginger "mother":
- 1 cup water
- 7–10 tbsp. fresh grated ginger root
- white sugar (variable amount)
- 1 tsp. baker's yeast

For the pop:
- 1½ cups white sugar
- 6-inch piece fresh ginger root, grated (less for a weaker taste)
- 21 cups boiling water
- juice of 1 lemon

YOU WILL NEED
· COOKING THERMOMETER

MAKES & KEEPS
Makes just over 5 quarts.
Keeps at least 2–3 months.

METHOD
To make the ginger beer plant, mix the water with 1 tbsp. each of ginger and sugar in a screw-top jar.

Sprinkle in the yeast and cover with a cloth or lid. Keep it in a warm place (where you can see it; try also talking to it and inviting it to ferment). Add a little more sugar and ginger every day until it starts bubbling. After about 7–10 days it will be ready.

When you are ready to make the pop, strain the liquid off to use. The "gunk" left in your strainer is the ginger beer plant. Feed it with water, sugar, and ginger to keep it alive. After making a few batches, you can divide it and start one off for a friend.

In a large saucepan, add the sugar and ginger to the water and simmer for 20 minutes. Let cool to 80°F, then add the lemon juice and the liquid you strained off from the plant. Put into sterilized bottles immediately, leaving at least 3 inches at the top. Wait a couple of hours before you cork them (sometimes they explode, so choose a cork that can easily pop out).

The pop will be ready to drink in 7–10 days; it will have almost no alcohol content, but will be nice and fizzy.

— Variation —

LET FERMENT FOR 2–3 DAYS
LONGER FOR A STRONGER
ALCOHOLIC BEER.

Yarrow Beer

Adapted from Stephen Buhner's recipe

INGREDIENTS
- 5 lb malted barley
- 7 gallons water
- 3 oz. recently dried yarrow (or double the amount fresh)
- ¼–½ oz. brewer's yeast

YOU WILL NEED:
· COOKING THERMOMETER
· FERMENTING VESSEL

MAKES & KEEPS
Makes just over 6½ gallons.
Keeps 6–12 months.

METHOD
Preheat the oven to 150°F.

Mash the barley by coarsely crushing it and covering with 21 cups (just over 1¼ gallons) hot water, then place it in the oven for 90 minutes.

Next, strain the mixture, keeping the liquid, and "sparge" the mash—heat the remaining just over 6½ gallons of water and slowly let it drain through the barley mash. Collect all of it and mix with the first liquid.

Add half of the yarrow and bring to a boil. Let cool, then pour into a fermenting vessel with the yeast. Put the other half of the yarrow into a cheesecloth bag and hang it in the fermenter. Let it ferment until it is finished (normally 5–7 days), then bottle and cap—at this stage the alcohol content will be negligible. Let it ferment in the bottles. After 2 weeks, it will be ready to drink.

— Variation —

YOU CAN ALSO MAKE THIS AS FOR GINGER POP (P.169) AND DANDELION & BURDOCK (P.168)—THE LONGER YOU LET IT FERMENT (FROM 7–21 DAYS), THE STRONGER IT GETS.

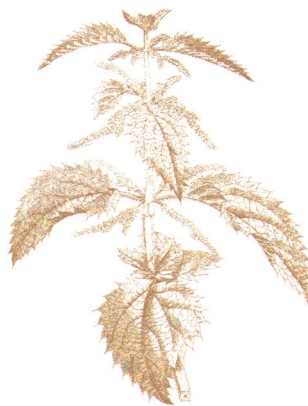

Nettle Beer

Courtesy of Susun Weed

A delightful drink that can be taken as a medicine for joint pain.

INGREDIENTS
- 2½ cups raw sugar
- juice and peel of 2 lemons
- 3 tbsp. + 1 tsp. cream of tartar
- 2¼ lb. fresh chopped nettles
- 21 cups water
- 1 oz. fresh yeast

MAKES & KEEPS
Makes just over 5 quarts.
Keeps at least 2–3 months.

METHOD
Put the sugar, lemon peel (no pith), lemon juice, and cream of tartar into a large casserole dish with a lid. Cook the nettles in the water for 15 minutes. Strain into the casserole and stir well. When it cools to lukewarm, dissolve the yeast in a little water and add to your casserole.

Cover with several folds of cloth and let brew for 3 days. Strain out the sediment and bottle. It will be ready to drink in 8 days.

Elderflower Champagne

INGREDIENTS

- 🍃 I lemon
- 🍃 I¾ cups white sugar
- 🍃 I tbsp. wine vinegar
- 🍃 12 fresh elderflower heads
- 🍃 19 cups boiling water
- 🍃 9½ cups cold water

MAKES & KEEPS

Makes just over 2 quarts.
Keeps up to 12 months.

METHOD

In a scrupulously clean large bowl, add the juice and zest of ½ lemon, and add the other half, sliced. Add the sugar, vinegar, and flowers. Bruise with a potato masher. Add the boiling water and stir for several minutes. Let sit for I–2 hours, then add the cold water, cover with cloth, and let sit for 2–4 days. Strain through cheesecloth and bottle it with corks.

Store for 7–10 days before drinking.

Dandelion Champagne

INGREDIENTS

- 🍃 4 cups fresh dandelion flowers, stems removed, fully opened
- 🍃 19 cups boiling water
- 🍃 I¾ cups white sugar
- 🍃 juice of 2 lemons
- 🍃 I tbsp. wine vinegar
- 🍃 9½ cups cold water

MAKES & KEEPS

Makes just under 7 quarts.
Keeps 6–12 months.

METHOD

Cover the flowers with the boiling water. Mix in the sugar and let sit for 12 hours. Strain and add the lemon juice, vinegar, and cold water.

Bottle, cork, and let brew (10 days for a nonalcoholic beverage drink and 3–4 weeks for a mildly alcoholic version).

Dandelion Coffee

Courtesy of Annie Powell

A delicious and healthy alternative to coffee.

INGREDIENTS

Dandelion roots, as many 2-inch long roots as you can find, scrubbed, chopped, and dried for 24 hours by a radiator

Place the roots in a single layer on a baking sheet in the oven at the lowest temperature. Cook slowly for 2–5 hours (depending upon the temperature of your oven) until the roots look charred, dark brown or black, and withered. Let cool thoroughly for I–2 hours. Store in jars until use.

KEEPS

Roasted roots will keep up to a year in an airtight container.
Once brewed, drink immediately.

METHOD

Put a saucepan of water on to heat. Add some dried dandelion root (about 3 pieces should be enough for a cup). Bring to a boil and simmer for 10–15 minutes. By this time, the water will be dark brown. Strain into cups and drink, adding milk and sugar to taste, if required.

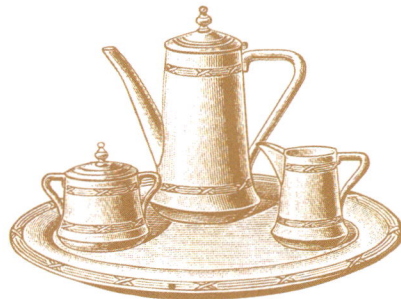

RECREATIONAL TINCTURES

"Recreational" tinctures are tinctures that have been sweetened with sugar or honey to make a tasty alcoholic drink. They are all made as for ordinary tinctures by mixing the ingredients and letting them steep for some weeks, then straining and bottling (pp.18–19).

The following recipes will make almost 3 cups and keep for years—though they are so nice they are unlikely to be given the chance. You can drink them undiluted in small glasses, mixed with sparkling water to make a refreshing drink, or made into a hot punch, mixed with boiling water.

Pear & Nutmeg Brandy

This is one of my most popular drinks, because it is absolutely gorgeous.

INGREDIENTS
- 4–5 pears, cut up
- 2 whole nutmegs, freshly grated
- 3 cups brandy (the best you can afford)
- 2 tbsp. honey

METHOD
See introduction and key techniques section (left and pp.18–19).

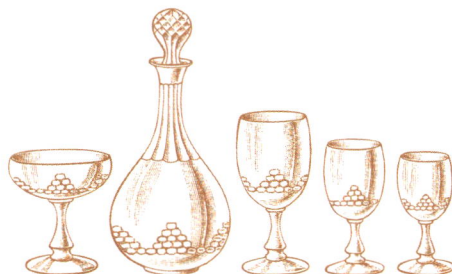

Aphrodisiac Brandy

INGREDIENTS
- 4 oz. dried ground ginseng root
- 4 oz. dried ground rhodiola rosea powder
- 4 cinnamon sticks, broken up
- 4 whole vanilla beans
- 2–6 whole chilies (depends on taste, because they will be hot)
- 3 cups brandy
- 2 tbsp. honey

METHOD
See introduction and key techniques section (left and pp.18–19).

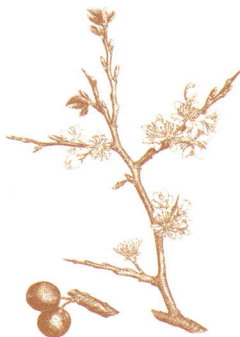

Sloe Vodka

Courtesy of Lynn Amanda Brown

A variation on the traditional sloe gin.

INGREDIENTS
- about 3 cups fresh sloes
- 3 cups vodka
- 1¾ cups white distilled sugar

METHOD
See introduction and key techniques section (left and pp.18–19).

Plum Mead

- 4 generous handfuls of fresh sweet plums
- 3 cups mead (honey wine)
- 1–2 tbsp. brown sugar
- 1–2 tsp. each ground cinnamon and nutmeg (optional)

METHOD
See introduction and key techniques section (left and pp.18–19).

Mabon Welcome Cup (Blackberry & Black Currant Brandy)

A Celtic tradition, the welcome cup was a special drink, often strong liqueur (with strong magic in it), offered to all at the start of a ceremony.

INGREDIENTS
- 1–2 large handfuls of fresh blackberries
- 1–2 large handfuls of fresh black currants
- 3 cups brandy
- 1 tbsp. honey

METHOD
See introduction and key techniques section (left and pp.18–19).

Very Berry Mead

A delicious and enjoyable drink, packed with vitamin C.

INGREDIENTS

1 generous handful of each of these fresh fruits:
- raspberries
- rowan berries
- hawthorn berries
- blackberries
- bilberries (or blueberries)

- 3 cups mead (honey wine)
- 1 tbsp. brown sugar, dissolved in 2 tbsp. hot water

METHOD
See introduction and key techniques section (left and pp.18–19).

Horseradish Vodka

Good with tomato juice or try it straight as a shot with lime juice and salt to wake you up. It is also a medicine that helps to stimulate the immune system and the circulation.

INGREDIENTS
- 1 cup fresh grated horseradish
- 3 cups vodka

METHOD
See introduction and key techniques section (p.172 and pp.18–19).

If taking medicinally, take 1–2 tsp. 1–2 times day.

Gorse Liqueur

Gorse is uplifting and cheering.

INGREDIENTS
- 4 handfuls of fresh gorse flowers
- 1–2 tbsp. honey
- 3 cups half and half vodka and mead mixed

METHOD
See introduction and key techniques section (p.172 and pp.18–19).

Drink sparingly. Beware: It is strong.

Medicinal Port Brandy

Courtesy of ChaNan Bonser

This is delicious and, of course, highly medicinal … you can use it for coughs, bronchial issues, at the first sign of a cold or flu; you can have little sips, mix with honey to taste, and also serve warm if you like.

INGREDIENTS
- 2 cups freshly picked elderberries
- 2 cups port wine
- 2 cups brandy
- 2 cinnamon sticks
- 1 tsp. dried ginger (or about 1 inch of fresh ginger root)
- 6 cardamom pods
- 8 black peppercorns
- 8 cloves

MAKES & KEEPS
Makes about 4 cups.
Keeps at least 2–3 years.

METHOD
See introduction and key techniques section (p.172 and pp.18–19).

— *Tip* —

ADJUST THE SPICES TO YOUR TASTE, ADDING MORE OR LESS AS YOU DESIRE.

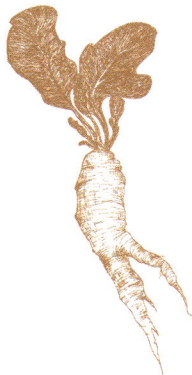

Swiss Gentian Aperitif Wine

Courtesy of Christine Herren-Valette

This fortified wine is good as both an aperitif (a predinner drink) and a digestive (taken after the meal). Gentian is an excellent liver stimulant that aids digestion. Yellow gentian is a digestive, reduces fever, and is a general tonic.

INGREDIENTS
- ¾ cup coarsely chopped fresh root of yellow gentian
- I cup apple schnapps (60 proof)
- 2½ (I-liter) bottles white wine
- zest of I lemon
- zest of 2 oranges
- ½ cup water
- 3 cups white distlled sugar

MAKES & KEEPS
Makes just over 3 quarts.
Keeps I year.

METHOD
Mix the chopped gentian root and apple schnapps. Cover and let macerate for 48 hours. Then add the white wine and the lemon and orange zest and replace the cover.

Let sit for IO days in a dark place, stirring a little every 2 days.

After IO days, strain and press through cheesecloth. Make a syrup (pp.21–22) by boiling the water and sugar together for I minute.

Mix the syrup and gentian wine and bottle.

— Tip —

THERE IS OFTEN A DEPOSIT ON THE SURFACE OF THE GENTIAN WINE, BUT DO NOT THROW AWAY. JUST STIR OR SHAKE THE BOTTLE TO REMIX AS IT IS DELICIOUS.

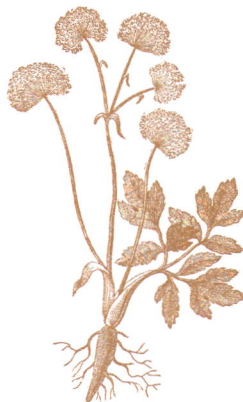

Angelica Archangel After-Dinner Liqueur

Courtesy of Christine Herren

INGREDIENTS
- 2 cups fresh angelica stems, cut to ½ inch in length (wash and dry with a dish towel after picking)
- 3 cloves
- 2 quarts + ½ cup apple liquor (40 proof)
- I¾ cups water
- 2 cups + 2 tbsp. white sugar

MAKES & KEEPS
Makes about 2½ quarts.
Keeps 5 years.

METHOD
Put the chopped angelica stems, cloves, and apple liquor in a large glass bottle. Let rest covered in a dark place for 2 months. Strain and press.

Make a syrup (pp.21–22) by boiling the water and sugar together for I minute.

Mix this with the angelica liquid and then pour into bottles.

HOMEMADE WINE

Wine can be made from anything edible. Whatever kind of wine you choose to make, the flowers/leaves/fruits should be at their prime and picked on a dry, preferably sunny day and placed in plastic liquid measuring cups. The following simple method, kindly given by Annie Powell, uses no chemicals or additives, other than wine yeast, and can be used for all the wine recipes here.

YOU WILL NEED

- LARGE PLASTIC PAIL OR CERAMIC CASSEROLE DISH
- CARBOY, RUBBER STOPPER, AND AIRLOCK (MUST BE THOROUGHLY CLEAN: SIMMER THE AIRLOCK AND RUBBER STOPPER FOR 5 MINUTES, RINSE AND PUT CLEAN WATER IN THE AIRLOCK)
- PLASTIC FUNNEL
- COTTON CHEESECLOTH (BIG ENOUGH TO COVER MOUTH OF PAIL/CASSEROLE DISH, WITH 3-INCH OVERLAP ALL ROUND
- STRING (ENOUGH TO GO AROUND MOUTH OF PAIL/CASSEROLE DISH WITH 6 INCHES EXTRA)
- BOTTLE BRUSH
- BLACK GARBAGE BAG
- SYPHON TUBE

MAKES & KEEPS
Each recipe makes just under 5 quarts, and can keep for years.

METHOD
Put the flowers or leaves into the pail or casserole dish.

Boil half of the water and pour it over them. Add the lemon juice and cover the pail with cheesecloth tied with string. Let sit for 3 days, shaking or stirring several times a day.

Boil the remaining water with the sugar. Add to the infused flowers or leaves and stir. Let cool until lukewarm, then add the yeast. Let sit for 1 hour.

Stir and strain the mixture through the cotton cheesecloth into the carboy, using a funnel (this is a two-person job) and fit the rubber stopper and airlock. Put the carboy into a black garbage bag (which keeps it warm and dark). Let sit in a warm place.

Within 24 hours (sometimes within minutes) it should start "blipping" (fermenting). If it hasn't within 24 hours, give it a shake. If nothing happens after another hour or 2, add another 1 tsp. yeast. Different wines ferment at different rates; when it has stopped "blipping" for a couple of weeks, syphon off into a clean carboy or bottles. Let sit at least 3 months before drinking.

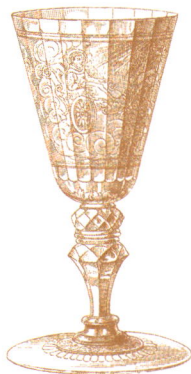

Gorse Wine

Courtesy of Annie Powell

To pick gorse flowers, grasp them between your thumb and index finger and pull. Only the yellow flowers are used, none of the green, and watch out for the spikes.

INGREDIENTS
- 1 gallon water
- 4 cups fresh gorse flowers
- juice of 2 lemons
- 4 cups granulated sugar
- 1 rounded tsp. wine yeast

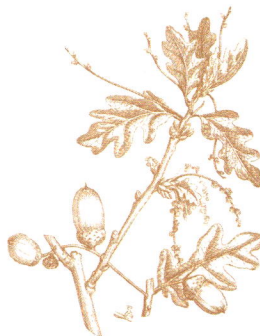

Walnut Leaf Wine

Courtesy of Annie Powell

INGREDIENTS
- 1 gallon water
- 3 good sprigs of fresh walnut leaves, crushed gently by hand
- juice of 2 lemons
- 4 cups granulated sugar
- 1 rounded tsp. wine yeast

Elderflower Wine

A favorite wine, perfect to make hay fever and cough medicine tinctures from.

INGREDIENTS
- 1 gallon water
- 8 cups elderflowers
- juice of 2 lemons
- 4 cups granulated sugar
- 1 rounded tsp. wine yeast

Oak Leaf Wine

Makes a good medium-dry white.

INGREDIENTS
- 1 gallon water
- 21 cups fresh oak leaves
- juice of 2 lemons
- 4 cups granulated sugar
- 1 rounded tsp. wine yeast

Ashwagandha Night Cap

Courtesy of Anne McIntyre

Ashwagandha is a wonderful Ayurvedic herb with deeply relaxing and stress-busting properties.

INGREDIENTS
- 1 tsp. ashwagandha powder
- 1 mug warm almond milk
- 1 tsp. rosewater
- pinch of cardamom powder

MAKES & KEEPS
Makes 1 mug.
Drink fresh.

METHOD
Warm the ingredients together.
Sip before bedtime for a restful sleep.

BEAUTY, BALMS & PERSONAL CARE

You can make your own all-natural beauty- and personal-care products that rely on the wonderful power of plants—from cleanser to lipstick to body butter, from soap and shampoo to shaving cream and deodorant. These preparations contain pure ingredients that enhance your health and feed and nourish your skin. Treat yourself and care for the environment at the same time.

Cleopatra's Cleanser

Courtesy of Teri Evans

Great for makeup removal. This is based on a recipe used by Cleopatra—she wouldn't have had grapefruit seed extract, but she would have had donkey milk …

INGREDIENTS
- 3 tbsp. + I tsp. olive oil
- 8 tsp. aloe vera gel
- 2 tbsp. rosewater
- 4 drops rose essential oil
- 2 drops grapefruit seed extract

MAKES & KEEPS
Makes ½ cup.
Keeps 6 months.

METHOD
Whisk the olive oil into the aloe vera. Continue whisking while you gradually add the rosewater. Add the rose essential oil and grapefruit seed extract and whisk well. Pour or spoon into a jar.

Massage into your face and neck twice daily. Either wash off with a facecloth (then tone and moisturize) or remove with cotton balls (then it will act as a moisturizer, too).

Mint Chocolate Face Pack

Courtesy of Teri Evans

Deeply cleansing, like all face masks, and really plenty of fun. It smells divine—almost good enough to eat.

INGREDIENTS
- I½ tbsp. raw cocoa powder
- I tbsp. white kaolin clay powder
- ½ cup dried peppermint leaves
- up to ¼ cup coconut oil

MAKES & KEEPS
Makes almost I cup.
Keeps up to 6 months in a jar.

METHOD
Mix the dry ingredients together. Gradually add the oil until you have a thick paste.

Apply to cleansed skin and then keep on for 15–20 minutes. Wash off well and moisturize.

— Variation —

YOU CAN SUBSTITUTE COCONUT MILK FOR THE COCONUT OIL AND REPLACE DRIED HERBS WITH THE SAME QUANTITY OF FRESH IF YOU WILL BE USING IT IMMEDIATELY.

Soothing Face Mask

Courtesy of Teri Evans

Suitable for all skin types, especially dry and irritated. These quantities will give you 2 applications—or share with a friend.

INGREDIENTS
- 3 tbsp. white kaolin clay powder
- 1½ tbsp. milk powder

Essential oils:
- 1 drop frankincense
- 1 drop chamomile

- 1 tsp. lavender water (possibly more)

MAKES & KEEPS
Makes 2 masks.
Use immediately.

METHOD
Mix the dry ingredients together. Add the essential oils and lavender water and stir well. Let sit for a few minutes, and then, if necessary, add more lavender water until you have a consistency that is easy to spread.

Use as described for Mint Chocolate Face Pack (opposite).

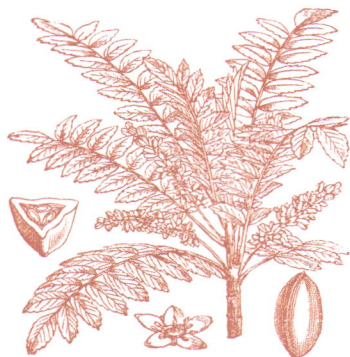

Nourishing & Cleansing Face Mask

Courtesy of ChaNan Bonser

A supersimple recipe, ready in an instant. Suitable for all skin types.

INGREDIENTS
- splash of rosewater
- splash of witch hazel
- 1½ tsp. chickpea (besan) flour

MAKES & KEEPS
Makes 1 mask.
Use immediately.

METHOD
Mix the rosewater and witch hazel with the chickpea (besan) flour to form a paste.

Use as described for Mint Chocolate Face Pack (opposite).

Yarrow Soothing Skin Wash

Courtesy of Maida Silverman

Yarrow makes an excellent astringent skin wash, especially suitable for oily skin.

INGREDIENTS
- 2 cups boiling water
- ½ cup dried yarrow flowering tops, crumbled

MAKES & KEEPS
Makes just under 2 cups.
Keeps in the refrigerator for 4–5 days.

METHOD
Pour the water over the yarrow flowers, let cool for 30–60 minutes, and then strain.

Pat it on the skin frequently to soothe irritation.

Lavender Toner

Courtesy of Teri Evans

This is a supereasy toner suitable for all skin types, especially blemished.

INGREDIENTS
- ¼ cup vodka
- ¼ cup lavender water (or rose, orange-flower, or other floral water as preferred)
- drizzle of vegetable glycerin
- 9 drops lavender essential oil

MAKES & KEEPS
Makes ½ cup.
Keeps 1 year.

METHOD
Pour all the ingredients into a bottle and shake well to mix.

Shake before use. Use daily, applying with cotton balls after cleansing. Avoid eye area.

Gentle Rose Toner for Mature Skin

INGREDIENTS
- just under ½ cup rosewater
- 1 tbsp. Rose Vinegar (p.165)
- 1 tsp. glycerin

Essential oils:
- 6 drops rose
- 6 drops rose geranium

MAKES & KEEPS
Makes ½ cup.
Keeps 6 months.

METHOD
Pour all the ingredients into a bottle and shake well to mix.

Use as for Lavender Toner (above).

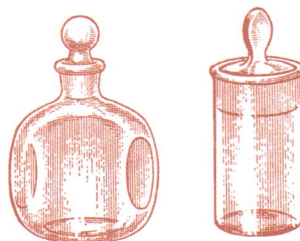

Wintertime Facial Toner

Courtesy of Jenny Pao

A facial toning elixir for all skin types. It soothes irritated skin, tightens pores, and keeps acne at bay.

INGREDIENTS
- 1½ cups water
- 1 peppermint tea bag
- 1 rooibos tea bag
- 1 chamomile tea bag

Essential oils:
- 1 drop rosemary
- 4 drops lavender

MAKES & KEEPS
Makes 1½ cups.
Keeps 2 weeks in the refrigerator.

METHOD
Bring the water to a boil, then let cool for 3 minutes. Pour the water over the tea bags in a pot and let sit for 5 minutes.

Cool completely before removing the tea bags. Add the oils and pour into a glass bottle.

Shake bottle before use. Apply toner daily to clean skin prior to moisturizing.

Medicinal Lavender Skin Tonic

Courtesy of Teri Evans

Suitable for all skins, the apple cider vinegar makes it especially good for problem skins. The smell does not linger once applied.

INGREDIENTS
- 2 handfuls of lavender flowers
- just under 1 cup Apple Cider Vinegar (p.165)
- just under 3 cups rosewater or Lavender Water (p.134)

MAKES & KEEPS
Makes almost 3¾ cups.
Keeps at least 1 year.

METHOD
Put the lavender flowers in the bottom of a large jar. Pour in the vinegar and rosewater and shake to make sure there are no air bubbles. Let it infuse for 1–2 weeks, shaking the jar occasionally. Strain through cheesecloth.

Shake before use. Apply daily after cleansing.

— Variation —

FOR A POWERFUL LOTION TO TREAT ACNE AND INTERTRIGO (A FUNGAL-TYPE INFECTION THAT CAUSES SORENESS IN SKIN FOLDS), ADD THESE ESSENTIAL OILS TO THE ABOVE LOTION:
- 100 drops/1 tsp. tea tree
- 100 drops/1 tsp. lavender
- 50 drops/½ tsp. thyme

APPLY THE LOTION 2–3 TIMES DAILY TO SORE AREAS.

Simple Rose Face Cream

Courtesy of Lynn Rawlinson

This is the simplest cream you can make.

INGREDIENTS
Oil fraction:
- ½ cup coconut oil
- 5 tsp. avocado oil
- 1 tbsp. honey

Water fraction:
- 5 tsp. rosewater

At the end:
- 10–15 drops rose (or rose geranium) essential oil (optional)

MAKES & KEEPS
Makes ¾ cup.
Keeps 6–12 months.

METHOD
Melt the coconut and avocado oils and the honey in a water bath, then gently warm the rosewater in a separate bowl in the water bath. Remove from the heat, and start to whisk the oil and honey mixture. As you do so, add a drop of rosewater.

Keep whisking and adding a little rosewater until you have used all of it, then whisk until the mixture starts to solidify. When it is semisolid, add the essential oils and whisk until well blended. Store in sterilized jars.

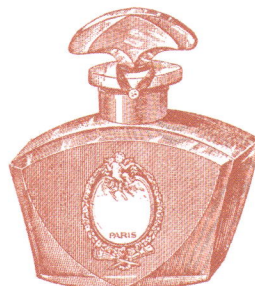

Rosy Lotion

Courtesy of Teri Evans

A nice, light lotion suitable as a face moisturizer for all skin types, including oily skin.

It is also good as a nongreasy hand nourisher for people who find hand creams too rich.

INGREDIENTS
- **just under ½ cup rosewater**
- **just under ½ cup glycerin**
- **50 drops/½ tsp. rose geranium essential oil**

MAKES & KEEPS
Makes 1¾ cups.
Keeps 6 months.

METHOD
Whisk all the ingredients in a bowl for a couple of minutes until they are blended. Then pour into a bottle.

Shake before use. Massage a small amount into your hands until absorbed.

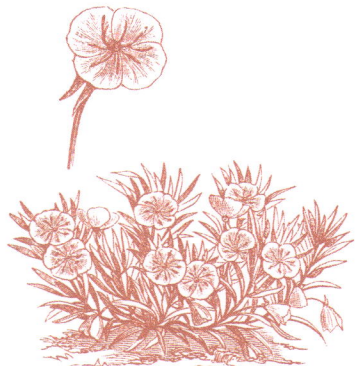

Antiaging Day Cream

Courtesy of Teri Evans

This has all the ingredients of a top quality, superexpensive skin cream from a laboratory. Carrot oil contains vitamin A, which helps to improve the elasticity of collagen and plump up your skin. Vitamin C is a free-radical scavenger—antioxidants help to slow down the effects of aging, basically reducing damage from UV rays. Rose helps to heal broken capillaries and reduces wrinkles, and glycerin to help hold moisture in your skin.

Creams can be difficult to make, so before starting, read the guidance on pp. 20–21.

INGREDIENTS
Oil fraction:
- **½ tsp. beeswax**
- **1 tsp. emulsifying wax**
- **2 tbsp. mango or shea butter**
- **1 tbsp. carrot oil**
- **1 tbsp. evening primrose oil**
- **½ tsp. vitamin C powder**
- **½ tsp. glycerin**

Water fraction:
- **5 tbsp. rosewater**

Extras:
- **10 drops rose essential oil**

MAKES & KEEPS
Makes about ½ cup.
Keeps at least 2–3 months.

METHOD
Gently heat together the waxes, mango or shea butter, and carrot and evening primrose oils in a water bath. When the waxes have melted, add the vitamin C powder and glycerin, and whisk well to mix.

Warm the rosewater to the same temperature. Whisk the rosewater into the oil fraction mix, adding the rose essential oil when the cream is cool.

Apply a small amount each morning to the face and neck.

Intensive Eye Serum

Courtesy of Monika Ghent

Oils can also be blended for different purposes. Use this eye serum for around the eye to treat dark circles or aging skin.

INGREDIENTS
- oil from 5 (400 IU) vitamin E capsules
- 1½ tsp. camellia seed oil
- 1½ tsp. rose hip seed oil
- 2 tsp. argan oil

Essential oils:
- 10 drops carrot seed
- 10 drops lemon
- 5 drops fennel
- 5 drops geranium
- 5 drops patchouli
- 5 drops rosemary
- 20 drops lavender

MAKES & KEEPS
Makes 5 tsp.
Keeps at least 6 months.

METHOD
Put all the ingredients into a dropper bottle and shake well.

Apply a few drops twice daily to the skin around the eyes.

Facial Serum for Sun-Damaged Skin

Courtesy of Monika Ghent

This serum of blended oils repairs sun damage at the cellular level.

INGREDIENTS
- 1½ tsp. camellia seed oil
- 1½ tsp. argan oil
- 1½ tsp. rose hip seed oil
- 1 tsp. jojoba oil
- oil from 5 (400 IU) vitamin E capsules
- 10 drops of liquid vitamin D

Essential oils:
- 25 drops lavender
- 10 drops lemon
- 10 drops carrot seed
- 10 drops palma rosa
- 5 drops rosemary
- 5 drops patchouli
- 5 drops geranium

MAKES & KEEPS
Makes 1-oz. bottle
(best to use pump spray dispenser).
Keeps 6 months in the refrigerator.

METHOD
Combine all the ingredients in a bottle and shake well.

Apply to the face 1–2 times daily.

Tropical Body Buff

Courtesy of Teri Evans

To exfoliate and nourish the skin.

INGREDIENTS
- ½ cup coconut oil
- 1¼ cups brown or raw sugar

Essential oils:
- 6 drops orange
- 4 drops lemongrass
- 3 drops ylang-ylang

MAKES & KEEPS
Makes up to 2½ cups.
Keeps 6 months.

METHOD
Warm the coconut oil in a water bath until it is just melted. Blend with the sugar well. Add the essential oils, making sure to mix well.

To use, massage a little into damp skin and wash off with warm water.

Caution
Do not use on damaged skin or on acne.

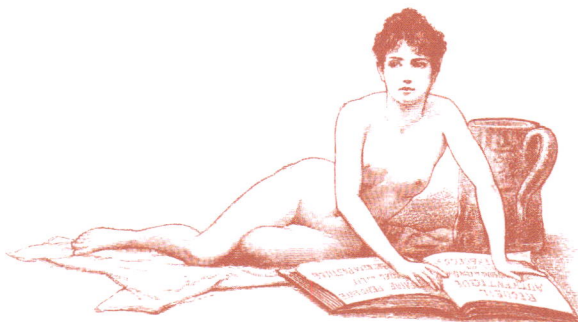

Choca-Coco Sugar Body Scrub

Courtesy of Monika Ghent

INGREDIENTS
- just under ½ cup coconut oil
- 1 cup whole cane sugar
- ¼ cup coconut sugar
- 2 tbsp. unsweetened cocoa powder
- 2 tbsp. jojoba oil
- 1 tsp. vanilla extract
- oil from 5 (400 IU) vitamin E capsules

MAKES & KEEPS
Makes 3 (½-cup) jars.
Keeps up to 1 year.

METHOD
Gently melt the coconut oil in a water bath, then blend with the rest of the ingredients in a mixing bowl before decanting into jars.

Use as for Tropical Body Buff (left).

Exfoliating Seaweed Scrub

Courtesy of Teri Evans

INGREDIENTS
- 1 tbsp. fine sea salt
- 1 tbsp. kelp powder
- 5 tsp. vegetable glycerin
- 7 tsp. sweet almond oil

Essential oils:
- 5 drops juniper
- 5 drops lemon

MAKES & KEEPS
Makes just under ½ cup.
Keeps at least 6 months.

METHOD
Mix the sea salt and kelp together. Add the glycerin and half the almond oil and mix well. If the mixture is too stiff, add more oil until it makes a thick, gloopy paste.

Add the essential oils and stir really well. Use as for Tropical Body Buff (opposite).

Note: Not suitable for dry skin.

Anticellulite Body Scrub

INGREDIENTS
- 1 tbsp. fine sea salt
- 1 tbsp. ground coffee
- 5 tsp. vegetable glycerin
- 7 tsp. sweet almond oil

Essential oils:
- 5 drops juniper
- 5 drops grapefruit

MAKES & KEEPS
Makes just under ½ cup.
Keeps at least 6 months.

METHOD
Make and use as for Exfoliating Seaweed Scrub (above), adding the coffee in place of the kelp.

— Tip —
IF YOU OMIT THE SEA SALT IN YOUR SCRUB RECIPES, YOU CAN USE THEM AS BODY MASKS INSTEAD. SPREAD OVER YOUR BODY, LET SIT FOR 20 MINUTES, AND THEN RINSE OFF.

Rosy Bath Bomb

Courtesy of Teri Evans

INGREDIENTS
- 2½ cups baking soda
- 2 tsp. rose hip oil
- 2 tsp. dry rose petals
- ¾ cup citric acid

Essential oils:
- 30 drops rose geranium
- 30 drops jasmine
- few drops red food coloring
- water in a spray bottle

YOU WILL NEED
· MOLDS FOR CUPCAKE-SIZE BOMBS

MAKES & KEEPS
Makes 12 bombs the size of cupcake liners (fewer if larger).
Keeps up to 1 year in an airtight container. (Note: They can't go off, but the smell slowly disappears as the essential oils evaporate.)

METHOD
Combine all the dry ingredients in a bowl and mix well. Mix the oils together, then add to the powders and mix again.

Add the food coloring to the water, then spray a little amount of water over the mix and blend in quickly and thoroughly. It has enough water added when you can squeeze it together and it only just holds together. Press firmly into molds. Let sit for up to 30 minutes to set, then turn out carefully.

Relaxation Bath Salts

Courtesy of Lucy Harmer

INGREDIENTS
- 3½ cups sea salt or natural kosher salt
- I oz. dried lavender flowers
- ⅔ oz. dried chamomile flowers

Essential oils:
- 21 drops lavender
- 21 drops chamomile

MAKES & KEEPS
Makes just over 4½ cups.
Keeps I year.

METHOD
Mix together and then keep in a sealed glass jar.

Add a small handful to your bath as required.

Love Spell Bath Salts

Courtesy of Lucy Harmer

I like to use Himalayan salt because it's naturally pink.

INGREDIENTS
- 3½ cups sea salt or natural kosher salt
- I oz. dried damascus rose petals

Essential oils:
- 14 drops damascus rose
- 14 drops geranium
- 14 drops palmarosa

MAKES & KEEPS
Makes 4½ cups.
Keeps I year.

METHOD
Mix all the ingredients together well and then keep in a sealed glass jar.

Add a small handful to your bath as required.

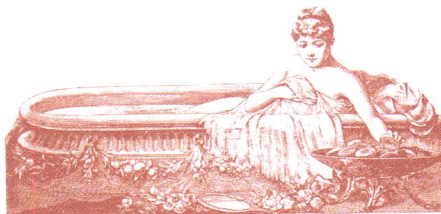

Purification Bath Salts

Courtesy of Lucy Harmer

INGREDIENTS
- 3½ cups sea salt or natural kosher salt
- 2 oz. dried lavender flowers

Essential oils:
- 20 drops lavender
- 10 drops rosemary
- 10 drops juniper

MAKES & KEEPS
Makes just over 4½ cups.
Keeps I year.

METHOD
Mix all the ingredients together well and then keep in a sealed glass jar.

Add a small handful to your bath as required.

Fruity Body Custard

Courtesy of Teri Evans

This light but deeply nourishing moisturizer is almost good enough to eat.

INGREDIENTS
- 2 tbsp. + 1 tsp. apricot kernel oil
- 1 tbsp. jojoba oil
- 2 tbsp. aloe vera gel
- 2 tbsp. orange-flower water

Essential oils:
- 10 drops sweet orange
- 3 drops pink grapefruit
- 2 drops bergamot

- 2 drops grapefruit seed extract

MAKES & KEEPS
Makes ½ cup.
Keeps 6 months.

METHOD
Whisk the apricot kernel and jojoba oils into the aloe vera gel. Gradually add the orange-flower water while whisking until the mixture thickens and becomes creamy. Add the essential oils and grapefruit seed extract.

Massage into the skin as required.

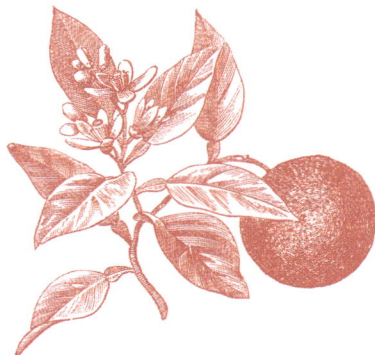

Invigorating Body Butter

Courtesy of Teri Evans

A rich body moisturizer (richer than Fruity Body Custard, left).

INGREDIENTS
- 2 tbsp. cocoa butter
- ¼ cup shea butter
- 2 tbsp. coconut oil
- ¼ cup evening primrose oil

Essential oils:
- 10 drops rosemary
- 10 drops lemon
- 5 drops ginger

MAKES & KEEPS
Makes 1 cup.
Keeps 6 months.

METHOD
Gently heat the cocoa and shea butters with the coconut oil in a water bath until they have melted. Remove from the heat and cool until lukewarm. Add the evening primrose oil and essential oils and whisk well.

The butter won't set at room temperature. For best results, put the bowl in the refrigerator, removing every 30 minutes or so to whisk. When nearly set, whisk well and pour into jars. Return to the refrigerator until finally set.

Luxurious Body Butter

INGREDIENTS
- 2 tbsp. cocoa butter
- ¼ cup shea butter
- 2 tbsp. coconut oil
- ¼ cup evening primrose oil

Essential oils:
- 10 drops jasmine
- 10 drops sandalwood
- 5 drops rose

MAKES & KEEPS
Makes 1 cup.
Keeps 6 months.

METHOD
Make as for All-Invigorating Body Butter
(p.187).

Antiseptic Body Butter

Good for skin prone to spots.

INGREDIENTS
- 2 tbsp. cocoa butter
- ¼ cup shea butter
- 2 tbsp. coconut oil
- ¼ cup evening primrose oil

Essential oils:
- 10 drops tea tree
- 10 drops oregano
- 5 drops thyme

MAKES & KEEPS
Makes 1 cup.
Keeps 6 months.

METHOD
Make as for All-Invigorating Body Butter
(p.187).

Revive Facial Mist

Courtesy of Monika Ghent

*A pick-me-up throughout the day, this also helps
to combat dry skin and uplift the spirits in winter.*

INGREDIENTS
- ¾ cup + 3 tbsp. still mineral water
- 2 tbsp. rosewater
- 1 tsp. glycerin
- 2 tsp. witch hazel

Essential oils:
- 6 drops spearmint
- 5 drops rosemary
- 3 drops palmarosa

MAKES & KEEPS
Makes 1 cup.
Keeps 1–2 months.

METHOD
Measure all the ingredients directly into
a spray bottle.

To use, shake well, close your eyes, and spray
onto your face.

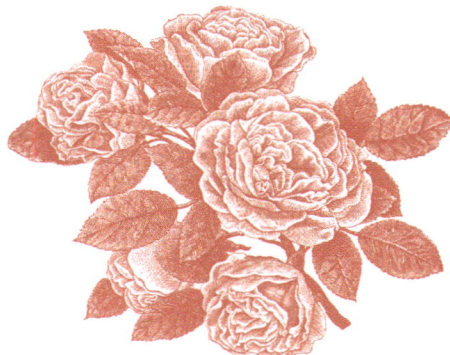

Lavender & Rose Hand Cream

Courtesy of Teri Evans

Creams can be difficult to make, so before starting, read the guidance on pp.20–21.

INGREDIENTS
Oil fraction:
- just under ½ cup coconut oil
- 2½ tbsp. beeswax
- 1 tbsp. cocoa butter

Water fraction:
- ¼ cup + 1 tbsp. rosewater
- ½ tsp. borax (see box, p.43)

Essential oils:
- 10 drops rose
- 8 drops geranium
- 5 drops ylang-ylang
- 15 drops lavender

MAKES & KEEPS
Makes nearly 1 cup.
Keeps 2–3 months.

METHOD
Heat the oil fraction ingredients together in a water bath, then remove from the heat and let cool slightly. Meanwhile, gently heat the water fraction until the borax dissolves.

Whisk the oil mix briskly until the bowl is lukewarm. Gradually add the water fraction ingredients without stopping whisking. Whisk as though your life depended on it. When the mixture looks creamy and white, add the essential oils while still whisking. You will notice a point when the cream starts to set; at this point, pour into jars.

Timing is the key with this recipe. If you wait too long, you will have to scrape the cream into the jars. If you pour it in too soon, the cream will separate.

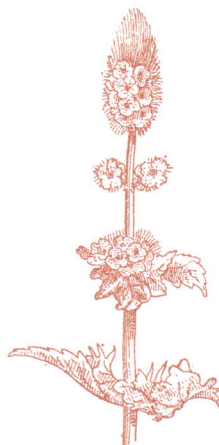

Antiseptic Hand Cream

INGREDIENTS
Oil fraction:
- just under ½ cup coconut oil
- 2½ tsp. beeswax
- 1 tbsp. cocoa butter

Water fraction:
- ¼ cup + 1 tbsp. lavender water or witch hazel
- ½ tsp. borax (see box, p.43)

Essential oils:
- 12 drops thyme
- 12 drops tea tree
- 12 drops oregano

MAKES & KEEPS
Makes nearly 1 cup.
Keeps 2–3 months.

METHOD
Make as for Lavender & Rose Handcream (left).

Nail & Cuticle Booster

Courtesy of Teri Evans

INGREDIENTS
- ⅓ oz. dried horsetail
- ¼ cup sunflower oil
- 3 drops lemon essential oil

MAKES & KEEPS
Makes about ¼ cup.
Keeps up to 6 months.

METHOD
Make an infused oil with the horsetail and sunflower oil (p.20). Add the lemon essential oil and bottle.

Massage a little oil into your cuticles at night to stimulate blood flow.

— *Tip* —

FOR A DEEP NAIL-STRENGTHENING TREATMENT, WARM THE OIL GENTLY IN A WATER BATH AND SOAK YOUR NAILS IN IT FOR 20 MINUTES. YOU CAN REUSE THE OIL AGAIN AND AGAIN.

Nourishing Nail Oil

Courtesy of Monika Ghent

Use this oil to strengthen and protect dry, brittle nails.

INGREDIENTS
- 2 tsp. jojoba oil
- 1 tbsp. sweet almond oil
- oil from 5 (400 IU) vitamin E capsules

Essential oils:
- 25 drops lavender
- 8 drops rosemary
- 6 drops spearmint
- 4 drops black spruce

MAKES & KEEPS
Makes 5 tsp.
Keeps around 6 months.

METHOD
Add all the other ingredients to a dropper bottle and shake well.

Apply 2–3 times daily to nails and nail bed.

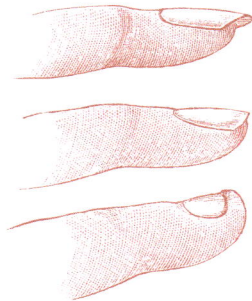

Foot & Leg Spray

Courtesy of Teri Evans

This helps to treat smelly feet, as well as to soothe and tone aching varicose veins.

INGREDIENTS
- just under ½ cup witch hazel
- 1 tsp. baking soda

Essential oils:
- 10 drops peppermint
- 8 drops rosemary
- 5 drops bergamot

MAKES & KEEPS
Makes just under ½ cup.
Keeps 1 year.

METHOD
Gently heat the witch hazel and baking soda until the baking soda is dissolved. Add the oils and store in a spray bottle.

Shake before use. Spray on your legs and feet 1–2 times daily.

Soothing & Refreshing Footbath

Courtesy of Johanna Herzog

This helps to protect against athlete's foot, and to treat aching and sweaty feet.

INGREDIENTS
- 2 handfuls of birch buds or leaves
- 2 handfuls of leaves and bark of ivy
- 4 cups boiling water

MAKES & KEEPS
Makes enough for 1 bath. Use immediately.

METHOD
Infuse the ingredients together for 10–15 minutes (p.15). Add to a basin containing enough hot water for a footbath; the water should be as hot as comfortable for the feet. Sit with your feet in it for 15–20 minutes.

"Beach Hair" Styling Spray for Curls

You can save a lot of money by making your own "beach hair" spray for that windswept look.

INGREDIENTS
- 2 cups boiling water
- 4½ tbsp. Epsom salts
- 1 tbsp. rosemary tincture (pp.18–19; use 1 tbsp. rosemary infused in 2 tbsp. vodka)
- 1 tbsp. lemon juice
- 2 tsp. aloe vera gel
- ½ tsp. almond oil
- 10 drops lemon essential oil (optional)

MAKES & KEEPS
Makes about 2 cups.
Keeps in refrigerator around 3 months.

METHOD
Mix the ingredients into a spray bottle and spray as much as is required to style your hair.

Citrus Hair Spray

This works well as a hair spray to keep hair in place, but only lasts for a week.

INGREDIENTS
- 2 lemons
- 1 lime
- 2 cups water (more if required)

MAKES & KEEPS
Makes 1 cup.
Keeps 1 week in the refrigerator.

METHOD
Cut up the lemons and lime. Simmer in the water for about 1 hour, keeping the water level up to 1 cup (half the amount you started with) by adding more as it boils away.

Let cool. Strain well and bottle in a spray bottle.

Spray as much as is required to style your hair.

Super Anticellulite Oil

Courtesy of Teri Evans

INGREDIENTS
- ¼ cup grapeseed oil
- 7 large fresh ivy leaves
- I tsp. wheatgerm oil

Essential oils:
- 7 drops juniper
- 3 drops geranium
- 2 drops rosemary

MAKES & KEEPS
Makes ¼ cup.
Keeps 6 months.

METHOD
Make an infused oil (p.20) with the grapeseed oil and the ivy. Add the wheatgerm oil and essential oils. Bottle.

Massage well into the usual problem areas 1–2 times daily.

Anti-Cold Sore Lip Balm

INGREDIENTS
- 2 tsp. cocoa butter
- 2 tsp. shea butter
- 2 tsp. beeswax
- 4 tsp. coconut oil
- 4 tsp. St. John's Wort Oil (p.83)
- oil from 5 (400 IU) vitamin E capsules
- 10 drops lemon balm essential oil

YOU WILL NEED
· 16 LIPSTICK MOLDS

MAKES & KEEPS
Makes 16 lip balms using lipstick molds.
Keeps 6 months or more.

METHOD
Melt all the ingredients except the vitamin E and lemon balm oils in a water bath. When melted, remove from the heat and add the vitamin E and lemon balm oil and pour into molds.

Chocolate Bomb Lip Therapy

Courtesy of Monika Ghent

This luscious lip balm heals and protects the delicate skin of your lips.

INGREDIENTS
- 2 tsp. beeswax
- 2 tsp. cocoa butter
- 2 tsp. shea butter
- ¾ oz. semidark chocolate
- 4 tsp. olive oil
- oil from 5 (400 IU) vitamin E capsules
- 10 drops peppermint essential oil

YOU WILL NEED
· 16 LIPSTICK MOLDS OR LIP BALM JARS

MAKES & KEEPS
Makes 16 lip balms using lipstick molds or jars.
Keeps 6 months or more.

METHOD
In a double boiler, melt the beeswax, cocoa butter, shea butter, and chocolate. When melted, add the olive oil, then take off the heat and add the vitamin E oil.

Finally, add the peppermint essential oil. Stir well and then put into the lip balm jars or lipstick molds immediately.

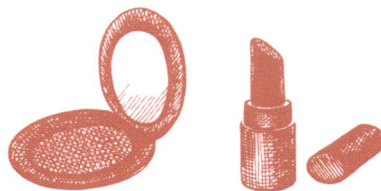

Doux-Baiser Lipstick (Sweet Kiss)

Courtesy of Christine Herren-Valette

Protects the lips while adding a touch of color.

INGREDIENTS

- 1 tsp. beeswax
- 4 tsp. Heal-All Marigold Oil (p.81)

Essential oils:

- 6 drops rose
- 12 drops rosewood
- tiny pinch of Italian ocher earth (pink)

YOU WILL NEED

· 5 OR 6 LIPSTICK MOLDS

MAKES & KEEPS

Makes 5 or 6 sticks. Keeps 1 year.

METHOD

Melt the beeswax and the marigold oil in a water bath. Remove from the heat and add the essential oils.

Mix all the ingredients with either a wooden stick (such as a wooden spoon handle) or a glass one (not metal or plastic) for 2–3 minutes.

Add the Italian ocher earth and stir for an additional 1–2 minutes to obtain a homogeneous color. Pour immediately into molds.

Beet Lippy

Vitamin-rich beet both conditions and colors your lips.

INGREDIENTS

- 4 tsp. St. John's Wort Oil (p.83)
- 1 tbsp. fresh grated beet
- 1 tsp. beeswax

Essential oils:

- 8 drops orange
- 8 drops lemon

YOU WILL NEED

· 5 OR 6 LIPSTICK MOLDS

MAKES & KEEPS

Makes 5 or 6 sticks.
Keeps 1 year.

METHOD

Pour the St. John's Wort Oil over the beet. Let sit in a covered jar for 3 days, then strain and squeeze out all the oil (wear gloves because the beet stains).

Gently melt the beeswax into the beet oil. Remove from the heat, stir the essential oils in thoroughly, and pour into molds.

Natural Mascara

Courtesy of Monika Ghent

This mascara isn't waterproof, so is easy to remove with water or vegetable oil.

INGREDIENTS

- 1 tbsp. white kaolin clay powder
- ¼ tsp. black mineral oxide
- ½ tsp. vegetable glycerin
- 1½ tsp. witch hazel
- 10 drops lavender essential oil
- 1 drop oregano essential oil

YOU WILL NEED

· A SYRINGE

· 2 WELL-WASHED MASCARA CASES

MAKES & KEEPS

Makes 2 mascara containers.
Keeps 3 months maximum.

METHOD

Blend all the ingredients well in a small bowl. Using a syringe, insert the mascara into the mascara container. Alternatively, store in a small jar and apply it with an old mascara applicator or eyebrow brush.

SOAP MAKING

You can buy the pure vegetable oil soap needed for many personal care and household cleaning recipes in this book or make your own from scratch. Making soap involves first preparing the lye, then separately warming and mixing an oil component, and finally mixing these. Other ingredients are mostly added later (unless the recipe says otherwise). The recipe for Citrus Oats & Honey Soap (opposite) explains the process in full; others refer back to it and explain the individual differences. Make sure you will not be disturbed, and keep children and animals away. Once underway, you cannot stop for some time.

Read "Key Techniques" on p.21 before commencing.

All these soaps will keep for several years.

Caution

Have all equipment ready before you start, including safety equipment. Soap making involves handling a dangerous chemical substance, so it needs extra caution. It helps to weigh or measure all the ingredients before you start, and have them safely stowed and ready to use.

YOU WILL NEED

· SAFETY: OVERALLS, GLOVES, PROTECTIVE GLASSES OR GOGGLES, HAIR COVERING
· VINEGAR OR LEMON JUICE ON HAND (TO NEUTRALIZE POSSIBLE LYE BURNS)
· DIGITAL SCALES (ACCURATE WEIGHING/ MEASURING IS ESSENTIAL)
· STAINLESS STEEL OR ENAMEL SAUCEPAN, WITH A 3–4-QUART CAPACITY
· SILICONE OR STAINLESS STEEL SPATULA/SPOON
· SMALL STAINLESS STEEL/GLASS/PLASTIC BOWLS
· PAIL
· LIQUID MEASURING CUP

The recipes on pages 195 to 198 use a cold process. For cold-process solid soap making, you will also need:
· A CANDY THERMOMETER
· MOLDS—EITHER SILICONE SOAP MOLDS OR A LARGE MOLD THAT YOU WILL LATER CUT INTO BARS—FOR EXAMPLE, A WOODEN BOX LINED WITH PLASTIC

The recipes on pages 198 and 199 use a hot process. For hot-process liquid soap making, you will also need:
· A SLOW COOKER (ONE USED ONLY FOR SOAP)
· A HANDHELD BLENDER (ALSO CALLED AN IMMERSION BLENDER)
· 1 OR MORE CONTAINERS WITH TIGHT-FITTING LIDS TO STORE 1 GALLON SOAP

Citrus, Oat & Honey Soap

Courtesy of Emma Warrener

*The oats give texture and add a fantastic
exfoliant effect.*

INGREDIENTS

Lye:
- 10½ oz. sodium hydroxide
- 30 oz. water

Oils:
- 21 oz. coconut oil
- 26 oz. sunflower oil
- 25 oz. good-quality olive oil

Extras:
- 2 cups oats
- almost ½ cup honey
- 100 drops/1 tsp. lime essential oil
- 100 drops/1 tsp. lemongrass essential oil

MAKES

Makes about 30 bars, each weighing 3½ oz.

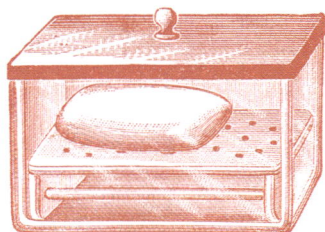

METHOD

Wearing gloves and eye protection, make the lye
by carefully pouring the sodium hydroxide
crystals into the container holding the water,
then put it safely out of harm's way to cool to
80.6–86°F. (Never pour water onto the lye.)

While it is cooling, gently heat the oils together
until the coconut oil is melted and cool to
80.6–86°F.

Carefully pour the lye into the oils and stir with
the spatula until you reach "trace"—this is when
you stir and the movement of the spatula creates
a line on the top of the mixture—a "trace" that
doesn't disappear. It's a sign that your soap has
reached full saponification—when the lye has
turned the oils to soap—and indicates your
misture is ready. To reach trace usually takes
about ½ hour, but soap has its own time scale
and it can take much longer! Make sure to stir
very thoroughly, all around the sides and the
bottom of the pan, and continuously.

When you've achieved a trace, it's time to
add the extras (oats, honey, and essential oils).
It is easiest to do this by putting a small ladle
of the mixture into a small bowl, mixing in the
extras, then adding this into the main mixtur
and stirring well to be sure they are distributed
evenly through the mixture.

Pour the soap into molds and put in a safe place,
away from children, for it to set for 24 hours.
After 24 hours, remove from the molds (wear
gloves, because the soap is still caustic) and put
it in a dry place to cure for 4–5 weeks.

— Tip —

MIXING THE OILS IN A SMALL
AMOUNT AS DESCRIBED IS EASIER TO
WORK WITH AND ENSURES THEY ARE
WELL BLENDED. IT ALSO MEANS YOU CAN
EXPERIMENT WITH DIFFERENT ESSENTIAL
OILS WITHOUT THE DANGER OF RUINING
YOUR WHOLE BATCH OF SOAP, BECAUSE
SOME WILL REACT DIFFERENTLY.

Bug Off!
Insect Repellent Soap

Courtesy of Tanya Smart

INGREDIENTS

Lye:
- 4 oz. sodium hydroxide
- 13 oz. water

Oils:
- 13 oz. coconut oil
- 10½ oz. olive oil
- 3½ oz. cocoa butter
- 2 oz. shea butter

Essential oils:
- 2 tsp. may chang
- 100 drops/1 tsp. Virginian cedarwood
- 100 drops/1 tsp. juniper
- 50 drops/½ tsp. basil

MAKES

Makes 12 bars, each weighing 3½ oz.

METHOD

Make as for Citrus, Oat & Honey Soap (p.195). First, prepare the lye and set aside to warm. Then warm the oils. Mix the lye and the oil parts together to trace, before adding the essential oils.

Sugar & Spice
Body & Shampoo Bar

Courtesy of Tanya Smart

INGREDIENTS

Lye:
- 4 oz. sodium hydroxide
- 13 oz. water

Oils:
- 13 oz. coconut oil
- 10½ oz. olive oil
- 3½ oz. cocoa butter
- 2 oz. shea butter

- 1 tbsp. golden syrup or light corn syrup
- 2 tsp. jojoba oil

Essential oils:
- 1½ tsp. orange
- 100 drops/1 tsp. ylang ylang
- 100 drops/1 tsp. black pepper
- 50 drops/½ tsp. ground cinnamon
- 50 drops/½ tsp. ground nutmeg

MAKES

Makes 12 bars, each weighing 3½ oz.

METHOD

Make as for Citrus, Oat & Honey Soap (p.195). First, prepare the lye and set aside to warm. Then warm the oils, adding the golden syrup to the mix as it is warming. Mix the lye and the oil parts together to trace, before adding the jojoba oil and essential oils.

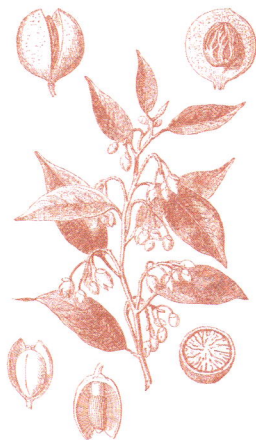

Gardeners' Soap for Dirty Nails

Courtesy of Tanya Smart

INGREDIENTS

Lye:
- 4 oz. sodium hydroxide
- 13 oz. water

Oils:
- 13 oz. coconut oil
- 10½ oz. olive oil
- 3½ oz. cocoa butter
- 2 oz. shea butter

Essential oils:
- 2 tsp. clary sage
- 100 drops/1 tsp. lavender
- 50 drops/½ tsp. rosemary
- 50 drops/½ tsp. bay

- 1 tbsp. coffee, coarsely ground
- 1 tsp. spirulina powder

MAKES

Makes 12 bars, each weighing 3½ oz.

METHOD

Make as for Citrus, Oat & Honey Soap (p.195). First, prepare the lye and set aside to warm. Then warm the oils. Mix the lye and the oil parts together to trace, before adding the essential oils, coffee grounds, and spirulina.

Baby Bubbles

Courtesy of Tanya Smart

Gentle and mild soap for sensitive skin.

INGREDIENTS

Lye:
- 4 oz. sodium hydroxide
- 13 oz. water

Oils:
- 13 oz. coconut oil
- 10½ oz. olive oil
- 3½ oz. cocoa butter
- 2 oz. shea butter

Essential oils:
- 2 tsp. may chang
- 100 drops/1 tsp. Virginian cedarwood
- 100 drops/1 tsp. juniper
- 50 drops/½ tsp. basil

- 4 tsp. dried lavender flowers
- 1 tbsp. dried marigold petals

MAKES

Makes 12 bars, each weighing 3 ½oz.

METHOD

Make as for Citrus, Oat & Honey Soap (p.195). First, prepare the lye and set aside to warm. Then warm the oils. Mix the lye and the oil parts together to trace, before adding the essential oils, lavender flowers, and marigold petals.

Luxury Soap

Courtesy of Tanya Smart

INGREDIENTS

Lye:
- 4½ oz. sodium hydroxide
- 13½ oz. water

Oils:
- 16¾ oz. coconut oil
- 10½ oz. olive oil
- 1¾ oz. shea butter
- 1 oz. beeswax

- 1 tbsp. milk powder (optional)
- 3 tbsp. honey
- 3 tbsp. oats

Essential oils:
- 100 drops/1 tsp. sandalwood
- 100 drops/1 tsp. frankincense
- 100 drops/1 tsp. rose
- 100 drops/1 tsp. ylang-ylang
- 50 drops/½ tsp. patchouli

- 2 tsp. castor oil

MAKES

Makes 12 bars, each weighing 3½ oz.

METHOD

Make as for Citrus, Oat & Honey Soap (p.195). First, prepare the lye and set aside to warm. Then warm the oils, adding the milk powder, honey, and oats as they warm. Make sure the beeswax is completely melted with the other oils. Mix the lye and the oil parts together to trace, before adding the essential oils and castor oil.

Pure Olive Oil Castile Soap

Pure castile soap is made from olive oil using a hot process (p.194). An extremely moisturizing, mild soap, it is kind on the skin.

INGREDIENTS

- 47 oz. organic olive oil

Lye:
- 30 oz. distilled water
- 9.39 oz. potassium hydroxide

- 80 oz. distilled water (separate from the lye)

MAKES & KEEPS

Makes just over 5 quarts of liquid soap. Keeps 1 year or more.

METHOD

Put the olive oil in your slow cooker and turn it on to its low setting.

Meanwhile, make the lye. Do this outside, if possible, or by an open window. Put the 30 oz. of water into a large, stainless steel saucepan. Put on goggles and gloves.

Pour the potassium hydroxide into the water carefully and slowly, without splashing. (Note: NEVER pour the water into the lye, because this is very dangerous.)

Next, pour the lye-water mixture slowly and carefully into the oil in the slow cooker. Stir it with a spoon that can take the heat. The oil will become cloudy.

Stir carefully without splashing, until you have the "trace" on the top, as with all soap making. You may need to stir for a long time—an immersion blender on slow can take from 5–10 minutes to 40 minutes or more—and, once started, you cannot stop.

When you have the "trace," put the lid on the slow cooker and let it heat (still on low) for 20 minutes. Every 20 minutes or so give it another stir and mix well; don't worry if it separates—this is normal. Stir well to mix, being careful because it is still corrosive.

Fairly soon the mixture will get too thick to stir with the blender, so use a spoon or spatula to stir instead. (It's handy to have both.) The mixture will start to resemble thick mashed potatoes and be difficult to mix. Continue to stir every 20 minutes, until the thick mixture is translucent but yellowish. It will take up to 12 hours, but the blended soap may be done in 4–5 hours. If you need to, turn off the slow cooker and go to bed for the night, resuming in the morning.

After 4–5 hours, test it by carefully dissolving 1 oz. of the mixture into 2 oz. very hot water in a clear glass container.

Stir it: If it turns milky or cloudy, it needs to cook for longer; if it is clear, it's ready.

When it is ready, carefully weigh the thick paste (wearing gloves) and put it into a large saucepan. Bring the same quantity of water by weight (16 oz. water to every 16 oz. paste) almost to a boil and pour on top.

Stir gently to dissolve. This can take a long time—you need to stir, possibly heat it some more, and stir again. If it keeps forming a whitish layer on top, you need to dilute more— add up to the same amount of water again and heat, stirring gently. Store in large jars.

Although I have used it immediately, it becomes more gentle with time, and I recommend letting it sit for 4–6 weeks to "cure" before use.

Liquid Castile Soap

Nowadays, many blended vegetable oil soaps are called "castile" or "Marseille" soap. This blended soap is less moisturizing but more strongly cleansing than the pure olive oil one.

INGREDIENTS
- 20 oz. olive oil
- 14 oz. sunflower oil
- 15 oz. coconut oil

Lye:
- 30 oz. distilled water
- 9½ oz. potassium hydroxide

- 80 oz. distilled water (separate from the lye)

MAKES & KEEPS
Makes just over 5 quarts of liquid soap. Keeps 1 year or more.

METHOD
Make as for Pure Olive Oil Castile Soap (left), replacing the single quantity of olive oil with the blend of 3 oils (above). These ingredients will take less time to saponify than the Pure Olive Oil Castile Soap, so you'll find you won't be stirring the mixture for as long.

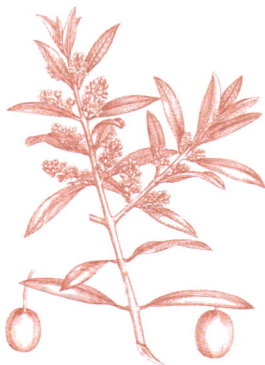

<<<<<<<<<<<<<<<<<<<<<<<<<<<<<<<<<<<<<<<<<<<<<<<<<<<<<<<<<<<<<<<<<<<<<<<<<<<<<<<<

Luxury Moisturizing Handwash

INGREDIENTS
- 2 tsp. avocado oil

Essential oils:
- 10 drops chamomile
- 10 drops lavender
- 10 drops neroli

- 1 tsp. glycerin
- 2 tbsp. liquid soap (Pure Olive Oil Castile Soap, pp.198–99, will be the most moisturizing)
- 2 tbsp. + 2 tsp. boiled or distilled water
- 2 tbsp. + 2 tsp. rosewater

MAKES & KEEPS
Makes ½ cup.
Keeps effective at least 3 months.

METHOD
Whisk the avocado oil and essential oils into the glycerin. Slowly mix in the rest of the ingredients. Pour into a hand-soap dispenser. Shake from time to time.

Lavender Handwash

INGREDIENTS
- 2 tsp. Lavender-Infused Oil (p.73)
- 30 drops lavender essential oil
- 1 tsp. glycerin
- 2 tbsp. Liquid Castile Soap (p.199)
- 2 tbsp. + 2 tsp. boiled or distilled water
- 2 tbsp. + 2 tsp. lavender water

MAKES & KEEPS
Makes ½ cup.
Keeps effective at least 3 months.

METHOD
Whisk the Lavender-Infused Oil and essential oil into the glycerin. Then make and use as for Luxury Moisturizing Handwash (above).

Mandarin Handwash

INGREDIENTS
- 2 tsp. infused lemon oil (p.20)

Essential oils:
- 20 drops mandarin
- 20 drops orange
- 10 drops tea tree

- 1 tsp. glycerin
- 2 tbsp. Liquid Castile Soap (p.199)
- 2 tbsp. + 2 tsp. boiled or distilled water
- 2 tbsp. + 2 tsp. orange-flower or witch hazel water

MAKES & KEEPS
Makes ½ cup.
Keeps at least 3 months.

METHOD
Make as for Luxury Moisturizing Handwash (left).

Antibacterial Liquid Handwash

This combines the bacteria–zapping actions of witch hazel, tea tree, lavender, and thyme to make a powerful soap with a fresh odor.

INGREDIENTS
- 2 tsp. almond oil

Essential oils:
- 20 drops tea tree
- 20 drops lavender
- 10 drops thyme

- 1 tsp. glycerin
- 2 tbsp. Liquid Castile Soap (p.199)
- 3 tbsp. + 1 tsp. boiled or distilled water
- 2 tbsp. distilled witch hazel

MAKES & KEEPS
Makes ½ cup.
Keeps at least 3 months.

METHOD
Make as for Luxury Moisturizing Handwash (left).

Moisturizing Working Hand Scrub

Courtesy of Teri Evans

INGREDIENTS
- 5½ tbsp. fine sea salt
- up to 6¾ tbsp. sunflower oil

Essential oils:
- 10 drops lemon
- 15 drops lavender
- 10 drops geranium

MAKES & KEEPS
Makes ¾ cup.
Keeps 6 months.

METHOD
Put the salt into a bowl and trickle enough sunflower oil into it to make a thick paste. Add the essential oils and stir well. Store in a jar.

Wet your hands and massage about 1 tsp. of the scrub gently into your hands. Rinse off. The oil should leave your hands feeling soft.

Clay Soap Alternative

A simple clay wash for your face, hands, body, and hair. Use any fine clay earth, such as Tilak from India or Rassoul Clay from Morocco, or whatever you have locally (if you dig up your own, be sure to carefully sift and filter it to remove pebbles).

INGREDIENTS
- 1–3 tsp. fine clay
- 1–3 tsp. rosewater

MAKES & KEEPS
1 wash.
Make and use same day.

METHOD
Wet your skin, take a little clay powder, and rub it over your skin, applying more water as needed. Let it stay on the skin for a few minutes, and wash off. For a lovely face wash, mix the clay with a little rosewater and then apply.

Psoriasis Skin Scrub

Courtesy of Lynn Rawlinson

Use this gentle alternative to soap in the bath or shower to help with descaling.

INGREDIENTS
- ½ cup coconut oil
- ¼ cup Lavender-Infused Oil (p.73)
- ⅓ cup oatmeal
- 25 drops/¼ tsp. helichynum essential oil

MAKES & KEEPS
Makes almost 1 cup.
Keeps 1 year.

METHOD
Melt the coconut and lavender oils in a double boiler or water bath. Let sit until it starts to cool. Whisk until it is lukewarm and the oil is starting to solidify. Blend in the oatmeal and add the essential oil.

Before bathing, apply skin scrub to a facecloth and lightly rub over the body. Soak in the bath or shower, rubbing the skin while in the water. Towel dry, leaving the skin soft and smooth.

Antiaging Skin Scrub

Courtesy of Lynn Rawlinson

INGREDIENTS
- ½ cup coconut oil
- ¼ cup Lavender-infused Oil (p.73)
- ⅓ cup oatmeal

Essential oils:
- 15 drops frankincense
- 4 drops geranium
- 4 drops neroli light
- 10 drops lavender

MAKES & KEEPS
Makes almost 1 cup.
Keeps 1 year.

METHOD
Make and use as for Psoriasis Skin Scrub (above).

Healing Skin Scrub

Courtesy of Lynn Rawlinson

INGREDIENTS
- ½ cup coconut oil
- ¼ cup Lavender-infused Oil (p.73)
- ⅓ cup oatmeal

Essential oils:
- ¼ tsp. lavender
- 10 drops geranium

MAKES & KEEPS
Makes almost 1 cup.
Keeps 1 year.

METHOD
Make and use as for Psoriasis Skin Scrub (p.201).

Coconut Scrub for Blemishes

Courtesy of Lynn Rawlinson

INGREDIENTS
- ½ cup coconut oil
- ¼ cup Lavender-infused Oil (p.73)
- ⅓ cup oatmeal

Essential oils:
- 30 drops lavender
- 10 drops chamomile

MAKES & KEEPS
Makes/almost 1 cup.
Keeps 1 year.

METHOD
Make and use as for Psoriasis Skin Scrub (p.201).

Soapwort Shampoo for Dark Hair

Courtesy of Teri Evans

This leaves your hair so soft and glossy you will love it!

INGREDIENTS
Dried herbs:
- ½ oz. Irish moss seaweed
- 1 oz. soapwort root, coarsely ground
- ½ oz. sage

- ⅔ cup boiling water

MAKES & KEEPS
Enough for 1–2 applications.
Use within 3 days.

METHOD
Crumble the Irish moss and mix in with the other dry ingredients. Put into a bowl and pour in the boiling water. Let cool stirring occasionally. Strain through cheesecloth, pushing it through to leave a greenish slime.

Use like normal shampoo, but don't expect it to foam. Rinse well.

Note: Avoid getting it in your eyes—it will sting a lot.

Soapwort Shampoo for Blondes

Courtesy of Teri Evans

INGREDIENTS
Dried herbs:
- ½ oz. Irish moss seaweed
- 1 oz. soapwort root, coarsely ground
- ½ oz. chamomile

- ⅔ cup boiling water

MAKES & KEEPS
Enough for 1–2 applications.
Use within 3 days.

METHOD
Make and use as for Soapwort Shampoo for Dark Hair (above).

Soapwort Shampoo for Redheads

Courtesy of Teri Evans

INGREDIENTS
Dried herbs:
- ½ oz. Irish moss seaweed
- 1 oz. soapwort root, coarsely ground
- ½ oz. marigold petals
- ⅔ cup boiling water

MAKES & KEEPS
Enough for 1–2 applications.
Use within 3 days.

METHOD
Make and use as for Soapwort Shampoo for
Dark Hair (left).

Red Clover Mild Shampoo

For normal hair, and also good for children.

INGREDIENTS
- 1 cup boiling distilled water
- ¼ cup fresh red clover flowers
  (or ¼ oz. dried)
- 1 tsp. apricot kernel oil or almond oil
- 2 drops Roman chamomile essential oil
- 2 tbsp. liquid soap, castile if desired
  (p.199), or any kind of shampoo base

MAKES & KEEPS
Makes just over 1 cup.
Keeps up to 2 months.

METHOD
Make and use as for Comfrey & Elder Shampoo
for Dry Hair (right).

Comfrey & Elder Shampoo for Dry Hair

Courtesy of Karen Stephenson

INGREDIENTS
- ¼ cup fresh comfrey root (or ¼ oz. dried)
- ¼ cup fresh elderflowers (or ¼ oz. dried)
- 1 cup boiling distilled water

Essential oils:
- 6 drops neroli
- 6 drops lavender
- 1 tsp. apricot kernel oil or almond oil
- 2 tbsp. liquid soap, castile if desired
  (p.199), or any type of shampoo base

MAKES & KEEPS
Makes just over 1 cup.
Keeps up to 2 months.

METHOD
Infuse the herbs with the boiling water for
20 minutes (p.15). Strain and mix the essential
oils with the apricot kernel or almond oil, then
mix thoroughly with the soap or shampoo base.
Gently mix with the infused herbs.

Shake gently before each use.

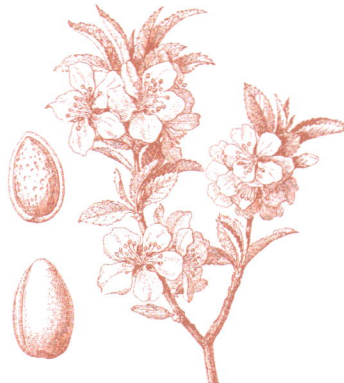

Willow Shampoo for Oily Hair

Courtesy of Karen Stephenson

INGREDIENTS

- 1 cup boiling distilled water
- ⅓ oz. dried white willow bark
- ⅓ oz. dried lemongrass (or ¼ cup freshly grated)
- 1 tsp. apricot kernel oil or almond oil

Essential oils:
- 6 drops bergamot
- 6 drops cedarwood
- 2 tbsp. liquid soap, castile if desired (p.199), or any kind of shampoo base

MAKES & KEEPS

Makes just over 1 cup.
Keeps up to 2 months.

METHOD

Make and use as described for Comfrey & Elder Shampoo for Dry Hair (p.203).

Burdock Antidandruff Shampoo

Courtesy of Karen Stephenson

INGREDIENTS

- 1 cup boiling distilled water
- ¼ cup grated fresh burdock root (or ¼ oz. dried)
- ¼ cup fresh chamomile flowers (or ¼ oz. dried)
- 1 tsp. apricot kernel oil or almond oil
- 12 drops rosemary essential oil
- 2 tbsp. liquid soap, castile if desired (p.199), or any kind of shampoo base

MAKES & KEEPS

Makes just over 1 cup.
Keeps up to 2 months.

METHOD

Make and use as described for Comfrey & Elder Shampoo for Dry Hair (p.203).

Cornstarch & Rosemary Dry Shampoo

A quick alternative to washing your hair.

INGREDIENTS

- 1 tbsp. dried rosemary, ground to a powder
- 1 cup cornstarch

MAKES & KEEPS

Makes about 1 cup.
Keeps at least a year if kept dry.

METHOD

Thoroughly mix the rosemary and cornstarch. Store in a sugar shaker for easy use. Apply a little of the powder to your hair roots. Rub it in well with your fingers, then brush it thoroughly to remove the grease.

— *Tip* —

ADD A COUPLE OF DROPS OF AN
ESSENTIAL OIL TO YOUR SHAMPOO
FOR A STRONGER FRAGRANCE.

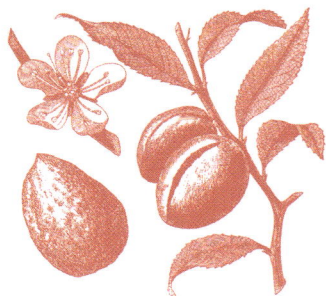

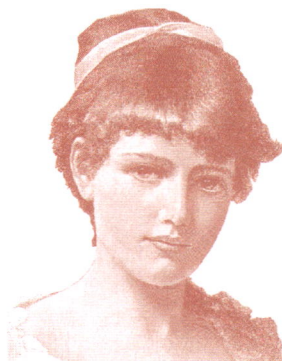

Nettle & Sage Shampoo for Graying Hair

Use this to slow down graying.

INGREDIENTS

- 🍃 I cup boiling distilled water
- 🍃 ⅓ oz. dried nettles
- 🍃 ⅓ oz. dried sage
- 🍃 I tsp. almond oil
- 🍃 4 drops rosemary essential oil
- 🍃 2 tbsp. liquid soap, castile if desired (p.199), or any kind of shampoo base

MAKES & KEEPS

Makes just over I cup.
Keeps up to 2 months.

METHOD

Make and use as described for Comfrey & Elder Shampoo for Dry Hair (p.203).

Hair Mud

Courtesy of Teri Evans

*Suitable for all hair types except very dry.
Either use it as a shampoo or leave it in for
20 minutes as a deep cleansing hair pack.
Your hair feels incredibly clean after use.*

INGREDIENTS

- 🍃 ½ tbsp. rhassoul mud powder (this is a Moroccan mud from the Atlas Mountains but you can use any kind of clay)
- 🍃 2 tbsp. herbal infusion (p.15): chamomile for blonde; marigold for red; nettle for brown; sage or black tea for black

MAKES & KEEPS

Enough for I–2 applications.
Keep in the refrigerator and use within I week.

METHOD

Mix the mud and herbal infusion well. Let it sit for 5 minutes. Stir again and add more infusion, if needed.

Massage the clay through your hair like a shampoo. Let sit for a few minutes, then rinse off thoroughly.

Orange, Lime & Grapefruit Conditioner

Courtesy of Emma Warrener

INGREDIENTS

Oil fraction:
- 1 tsp. coconut oil
- 2 tbsp. emulsifying wax
- 1 tsp. grapeseed oil

- ½ cup water (or floral water, or herbal infusion, p.15)
- 1 tsp. glycerin
- oil from 2 (400 IU) vitamin E capsules

Essential oils:
- 30 drops sweet orange
- 30 drops lime
- 30 drops grapefruit

MAKES & KEEPS

Makes just under ⅔ cup.
Keeps up to 1 year.

METHOD

Gently heat the oil fraction in a double boiler with the water (or floral water or herbal infusion) in the bottom pan. When the oils are melted, remove the pan from the heat and let cool for 5 minutes.

Meanwhile, measure the warmed water and top up to ½ cup. Add the glycerin to the water and stir thoroughly.

Slowly add the water mixture to the oil mixture, whisking continuously. The mixture will thicken up as it cools down. Once all of the water has been added, mix in the vitamin E oil and essential oils.

Let cool completely, whisking now and then to make sure that the liquid doesn't separate.

Store in a recycled plastic shampoo/conditioner bottle for ease of use.

Apply to clean, wet hair, leave in for 2–4 minutes, then rinse thoroughly.

Nit-Deterring Conditioner

INGREDIENTS

Oil fraction:
- 1 tsp. coconut oil
- 2 tbsp. emulsifying wax
- 1 tsp. neem oil

- ½ cup water (or lavender water or quassia infusion, p.15)
- 1 tsp. glycerin
- oil from 2 (400 IU) vitamin E capsules

Essential oils:
- 30 drops tea tree
- 40 drops lavender
- 20 drops thyme

MAKES & KEEPS

Makes just under ⅔ cup.
Keeps 1–2 months.

METHOD

Make and use as for Orange, Lime & Grapefruit Conditioner (left).

— *Variation* —

VARY THE ESSENTIAL OILS TO SUIT YOUR NEEDS. SEE THE HERBAL INFUSIONS AND OILS USED IN THE SHAMPOO RECIPES FOR INSPIRATION. IF YOU ADD AN HERBAL INFUSION IN PLACE OF THE WATER, THE CONDITIONER WILL KEEP ONLY UP TO 1–2 MONTHS.

— *Tip* —

PURE, PLAIN YOGURT IS A GOOD CONDITIONER. APPLY TO HAIR AS YOU WOULD A STORE-BOUGHT CONDITIONER. ONCE EVERY 1–2 WEEKS USE A DEEP TREATMENT, SUCH AS HAIR MILK OR OIL.

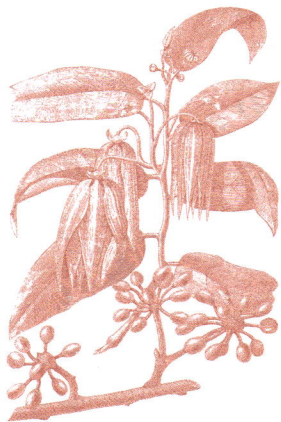

All-Natural Hot Oil Hair Treatment

INGREDIENTS
- 1 cup olive oil
- 3 tbsp. dried rosemary leaves

MAKES & KEEPS
Makes 1 cup.
Keeps 6 months.

METHOD
Make an infused oil with the rosemary and olive oil (p.20). Wash your hair and towel dry. Apply 2–5 tbsp. of the oil to your hair and massage it. Put a plastic cap on and wrap your head in a towel. After 45–90 minutes, wash your hair with a gentle shampoo.

Use weekly or less, as required.

Tropical Hair Milk

Courtesy of Teri Evans

This alternative to a hot oil treatment is less greasy but deeply conditioning for the hair. It smells deliciously tropical. Suitable for all hair types.

INGREDIENTS
- just under ½ cup coconut milk
- 7 drops lemon balm oil
- 4 drops ylang-ylang essential oil

MAKES & KEEPS
Enough for 1 application.
Use immediately.

METHOD
Combine all the ingredients in a bowl.

Massage into your hair and leave it in for 10–20 minutes. Wash with a gentle shampoo.

You can use this treatment up to once a week, as desired.

Sweet Rose Hair Oil

A sweet-smelling hair oil, simple to make.

INGREDIENTS
- ½ oz. dried rose petals or buds
- about 1 cup coconut oil
- 4–8 drops rose (or rose geranium) essential oil

MAKES & KEEPS
Makes about 1 cup.
Keeps 6–12 months.

METHOD
Put the roses and the coconut oil into a double boiler. Heat on low heat for 2–3 hours. Strain, add the essential oil, and pour into a jar.

Melt and use as described for All-Natural Hot Oil Hair Treatment (above). Alternatively, apply a little to your fingers and massage into the ends of your hair daily to moisturize.

Hair Growth Tonic

Courtesy of Johanna Herzog

*Helps to stimulate and warm the scalp,
so helping hair growth.*

INGREDIENTS
- 2 cups vodka
- ½ cup water
- 2 handfuls of fresh young birch leaves
  (collected in spring), shredded
- 2 handfuls of fresh nettle leaves and roots
- 1–2 fresh burdock roots, chopped
- I vanilla bean (optional)

MAKES & KEEPS
Makes about 2 cups.
Keeps 1 year.

METHOD
Mix in a covered jar and let sit for 2 weeks,
then strain as for any tincture (pp.18–19)

Dilute a little of the tonic with the same amount
of water and massage into the scalp daily.

Rosemary Vinegar

*Helps to promote hair growth as a hair rinse, and
to improve the memory and circulation as a drink.
It has a fresh smell and some antiseptic properties,
so is also useful in cleaning products.*

INGREDIENTS
- I cup rosemary flowering tops
- 2 cups Apple Cider Vinegar (p.165)

MAKES & KEEPS
Makes almost 2 cups.
Keeps at least 2 years.

METHOD
Make as for vinegars (pp.163–65).

For use on hair, dilute I part to 2 parts water.
Apply on wet hair after washing/conditioning as
a final rinse. You can also put it in a spray bottle
and spray on to wet hair.

Hair & Herbal Vinegars

*Herbal vinegars, when used as a hair rinse,
will encourage shine and help restore your hair's
protective acid pH. Different vinegars can be used
for different effect. Try nettle and rosemary for
promoting thickness and increased hair growth,
or rosemary and a few drops of tea tree oil to
treat dandruff, or sage to darken graying hair.*

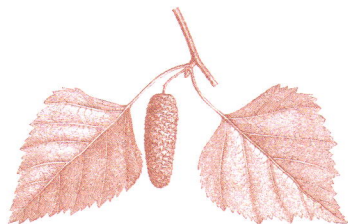

Teri's Tooth Powder

Courtesy of Teri Evans

A simple and effective tooth powder.

INGREDIENTS
- 1 tbsp. arrowroot
- 1 tsp. sea salt
- ½ tsp. baking soda
- 2 drops peppermint or cinnamon essential oil

YOU WILL NEED
- A MORTAR AND PESTLE

MAKES & KEEPS
Makes 4½ tsp.
Keeps at least 1 year.

METHOD
Mix the ingredients together well. Pound to a dry paste with the mortar and pestle and store.

Use as you would any toothpaste.

— Variation —

ADD 2 DROPS OF CLOVE OIL TO
THIS TOOTH POWDER FOR A STRONGLY
ANTISEPTIC EFFECT.

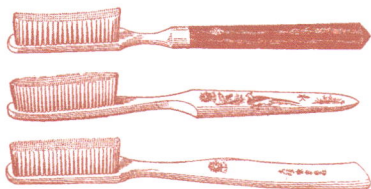

Cinnamint Toothpaste

Courtesy of Monika Ghent

To whiten the teeth and strengthen and heal gums.

INGREDIENTS
- 2 tsp. baking soda
- 2 tbsp. white kaolin clay powder
- 1 tbsp. arrowroot powder
- ½ tsp. vitamin C powder
- 1 tsp. ground cinnamon
- up to 1½ tsp. pure liquid soap (castile soap, especially Dr. Bronner's, is recommended)
- 15–20 drops peppermint essential oil

Tinctures (pp.18–19):
- 30–50 drops stevia
- 1 tsp. echinacea
- 1 tsp. sage
- 1 tsp. 3 percent hydrogen peroxide (naturally whitens teeth)

MAKES & KEEPS
Makes just under ¼ cup.
Keeps at least 1 year.

METHOD
Combine all the ingredients in a jar and stir well. Slowly add a little water to make a paste, and store.

Use as you would any toothpaste.

Medicated Tooth Powder for Gum Disease

INGREDIENTS
- ½ tsp. ground myrrh
- ½ tsp. ground cloves
- 4 tsp. baking soda
- I tsp. salt
- 3 tsp. chickpea (besan) flour

MAKES & KEEPS
Makes 3 tbps.
Keeps at least I year.

METHOD
Combine all the ingredients, mixing well.
Store in small airtight jars.

Use a small sprinkle, apply as any toothpaste.
Used daily, this amount could last I–3 months.

Medicinal Mouthwash & Gargle

*Helps to treat gum disease, mouth, and
throat infections.*

INGREDIENTS
Tinctures (pp.18–19):
- 4 tsp./20ml myrrh
- 4 tsp./20ml cloves
- 4 tsp./20ml peppermint
- 4 tsp./20ml sage
- 4 tsp./20ml horse chestnut

Essential oils:
- I drop lavender
- I drop geranium
- I drop eucalyptus

MAKES & KEEPS
Makes ½ cup.
Keeps 2 years or more.

METHOD
Mix the ingredients together in a bottle.

Shake before use. Dilute ½ tsp. in 2 tbsp. warm
water. Use to gargle or mouthwash twice daily.

Sage & Lavender Deodorant

Courtesy of Teri Evans

A floral scent that women may prefer.

INGREDIENTS
- 2 tsp. dried sage
- 2 tbsp. + 2 tsp. witch hazel
- 3 tsp. fresh cleavers (2 tsp. dried)
- I tbsp. vodka
- I tsp. benzoin tincture (Friar's Balsam)

Essential oils:
- 5 drops sage
- 5 drops lavender

YOU WILL NEED
· 2-FL.-OZ. SPRAY BOTTLE

MAKES & KEEPS
Makes almost ¼ cup.
Keeps 3–6 months.

METHOD
Let the sage infuse in the witch hazel for
2 weeks, and the cleavers infuse in the vodka
for 2 weeks (p.18). Strain and press both, then
combine. Add all the other ingredients and mix
in a bottle with a spray top. Shake well.

Shake before use and use as a normal
deodorant. Men may prefer it without the
lavender; simply add sage oil in place of
the lavender.

Citrus Fresh Deodorant

Courtesy of Teri Evans

A fresh smell that men may prefer.

INGREDIENTS
- 2 tsp. dried sage
- 2 tbsp. + 2 tsp. witch hazel
- 1 tbsp. fresh cleavers (2 tsp. dried)
- 1 tbsp. vodka
- 1 tsp. benzoin tincture (Friar's Balsam)

Essential oils:
- 5 drops lemongrass
- 5 drops tangerine

YOU WILL NEED
· 2-FL.-OZ. SPRAY BOTTLE

MAKES & KEEPS
Makes just under ¼ cup.
Keeps 3–6 months.

METHOD
Make as for Sage & Lavender Deodorant (opposite).

Sandalwood Deodorant

Courtesy of Teri Evans

A musky and sexy fragrance for men and women.

INGREDIENTS
- 2 tsp. dried sage
- 2 tbsp. + 2 tsp. witch hazel
- 1 tbsp. fresh cleavers (2 tsp. dried)
- 1 tbsp. vodka
- 1 tsp. benzoin tincture (Friar's balsam)

Essential oils:
- 5 drops sage
- 5 drops sandalwood

YOU WILL NEED
· 2-FL.-OZ. SPRAY BOTTLE

MAKES & KEEPS
Makes just under ¼ cup.
Keeps 3–6 months.

METHOD
Make as for Sage & Lavender Deodorant (opposite).

Tea Tree & Lemon Deodorant Powder

INGREDIENTS
- 1 cup white kaolin clay powder
- ¼ cup baking soda
- 1½ oz. arrowroot

Essential oils:
- 20 drops tea tree
- 20 drops lemon

MAKES & KEEPS
Makes 1½ cups.
Keeps 1–2 years in an airtight container.

METHOD
Combine all the dry ingredients in a bowl. Slowly add the essential oils, stirring continuously. Sift the powder before storing.

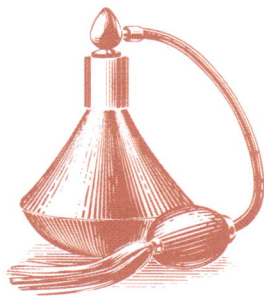

Lavender & Sage Deodorant Powder

Courtesy of Monika Ghent

This effective, body-friendly, underarm deodorant can also be used as baby powder. Men may prefer it without the lavender oil.

INGREDIENTS
- 4 oz. white kaolin clay powder
- ¼ cup baking soda
- 1½ oz. arrowroot

Essential oils:
- 20 drops lavender
- 20 drops sage

MAKES & KEEPS
Makes/1½ cups.
Keeps 1–2 years.

METHOD
Mix all the dry ingredients well in a bowl. Slowly drip in the essential oils, stirring constantly throughout. Sift the deodorant into a second bowl until all the powder has passed through the sifter.

You will be left with little balls of powder and essential oil. Using your fist, gently rub your hand around the sifter to break up these balls so that they pass through. Repeat the process two times. Then transfer the mixture into one or more glass jars.

Apply a dusting of the powder after washing and drying.

Luxury Shaving Cream for Women

INGREDIENTS
Oil fraction:
- ¼ cup sweet almond oil (or apricot oil or jojoba oil)
- 2 tbsp. shea butter or cocoa butter

Water fraction:
- 1½ cups spring water/filtered water
- 1 tsp. baking soda
- ¼ cup Liquid Castile Soap (p.199)
- ¼ cup honey
- ¼ cup aloe vera gel

Essential oils:
- 5 drops rose
- 5 drops jasmine

MAKES & KEEPS
Makes about 2 cups.
Keeps at least 3 months.

METHOD
Heat the oil and butter in a double boiler for a few minutes until it looks clear.

Remove the pan and let cool. Use the lower pan of the double boiler to heat. Gently heat the water, baking soda, and liquid soap. Stir until they are completely dissolved and mixed, then add the honey and aloe vera and mix in.

Slowly mix this mixture into the oils, a little at a time. Stir continuously.

Finally, add the essential oils and blend for a few minutes. Then let stand for a few minutes and blend again. Pour into jars.

Massage a little into the skin before shaving.

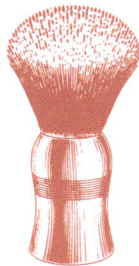

Moisturizing Shaving Cream for Men

INGREDIENTS

Oil fraction:
- ¼ cup sweet almond oil (or apricot oil or jojoba oil)
- 2 tbsp. shea butter

Water fraction:
- 1½ cups spring water/filtered water
- 1 tsp. baking soda
- ¼ cup Liquid Castile Soap (p.199)
- ¼ cup aloe vera gel

Essential oils:
- 4 drops pine
- 5 drops rosemary

MAKES & KEEPS
Makes about 2 cups.
Keeps at least 3 months.

METHOD
Make and use as for Luxury Shaving Cream for Women (opposite), adding the aloe vera when you would have added aloe vera and honey.

Tree Power Antiseptic Aftershave

This simple aftershave is antiseptic and strongly astringent.

INGREDIENTS
- 20 drops tea tree essential oil
- ½ cup distilled witch hazel

MAKES & KEEPS
Makes about ½ cup.
Keeps 1–2 years.

METHOD
Mix the ingredients and store.

Apply a little to skin after shaving.

Green Dragon Shaving Oil

Courtesy of Alaina Mecklenburgh

INGREDIENTS
- ⅓ cup almond oil
- 4 tsp. glycerin

Essential oils:
- 20 drops eucalyptus
- 20 drops lavender
- 50 drops/½ tsp. peppermint

MAKES & KEEPS
Makes just under ½ cup.
Keeps at least 6 months.

METHOD
Combine all the ingredients and store in a glass bottle.

Shake before use. Wet your face, put 5–6 drops on your hands, and apply to skin. Shave as usual.

Herby Aftershave

INGREDIENTS
- 2 tbsp. rosemary leaves (fresh or dry)
- 2 tbsp. lavender flowers (fresh or dry)
- 2 tbsp. chamomile flowers (fresh or dry)
- ¼ cup spring water
- ¼ cup vodka
- ¼ cup witch hazel
- 1 tbsp. olive oil

MAKES & KEEPS
Makes almost ⅔ cup.
Keeps 6 months–1 year.

METHOD
Mix everything together except for the olive oil. Make a tincture (pp.18–19). After straining and pressing out the liquid, add the olive oil and bottle.

Shake before each use.

Splash a little onto the skin after shaving.

VARIOUS ODDITIES

Everything we need comes from plants—and some things we don't need, too. From ink to car wax and some weird and wonderful things in between, this section contains a miscellany of useful recipes I have concocted and gathered over the years.

❧

Blue-Purple Ink

INGREDIENTS
- 2 handfuls of ripe elderberries (or bilberries/huckleberries)
- ¼ cup vinegar
- ½ tsp./2.5ml benzoin tincture (Friar's Balsam) or myrrh tincture
- 5 drops thyme or rosemary essential oil
- I tsp. gum arabic

MAKES & KEEPS
Makes about ¼ cup.
Keeps around 6 months.

METHOD
Simmer the berries in the vinegar, mashing with a potato masher and stirring to prevent them from burning, for 15 minutes. Strain and press through cheesecloth to get all the juice out (wear gloves because this juice seriously stains).

Mix the other ingredients with the dye/vinegar mixture and bottle.

Use the ink for painting or for writing with a dipping pen and inkwell.

Brown Ink

Courtesy of Teri Evans

INGREDIENTS
- 6–8 whole walnuts, gathered from the ground when blackened with age
- ½ cup water
- ½ cup vinegar
- I tsp./5ml benzoin tincture (Friar's Balsam) or myrrh tincture
- 5 drops thyme or rosemary essential oil
- I tsp. gum arabic for each ¼ cup of dye

MAKES & KEEPS
Makes about ¼ cup.
Keeps up to I year.

METHOD
Simmer the walnut in just enough water to cover for 30 minutes–I hour, topping up with the vinegar as the water boils away. You should end up with ¼–½ cup of dark brown liquid.

Strain the liquid and press through cheesecloth (use gloves and be careful, because this dye will seriously stain). Mix the other ingredients with the liquid and bottle.

Use as for Blue-Purple Ink (left).

Rose Petal Beads

Courtesy of Kamala Todd

The original Rosary prayer beads.

INGREDIENTS

- 10½ cups fresh, fragrant rose petals
- spring water (variable amount)

YOU WILL NEED

- IRON POT OR CAULDRON

KEEPS

Well-made beads can last more than 100 years.

METHOD

Put the rose petals into a little spring water in the iron cauldron and cover with a lid. Gently simmer (never boil hard or the essential oils will be lost) for 5 hours a day for up to 5 days. Add more water as required to stop the rose petals from drying out or burning.

Strain and press the liquid through cheesecloth to leave a thick, smooth, black paste. Roll the paste into bead shapes, using your hands (they shrink to one-quarter to one-half of the size when dry).

Place the beads on a plate and let sit in a dry, warm place (away from direct sunlight) for 5–10 days to dry. Roll each day to get a dense, smooth, round bead. Before they are completely dry, push a thick needle through the middle.

Store fully dried beads in glass jars. Do not let the beads get wet.

Waterproofing Mix for Canvas

Courtesy of Teri Evans

INGREDIENTS

- 1 cup soy, grapeseed or almond oil
- ½ cup turpentine

MAKES & KEEPS

Makes 1½ cups.
Keeps at least 1 year.

METHOD

Mix together and store in a cool place.

To waterproof, paint 2–3 coats on to dry canvas.

Lemon Boot Polish

Courtesy of Tony Haslegrave

INGREDIENTS

- 5 tsp. beeswax
- ¼ cup + 2 tsp. turpentine
- 1 tbsp. linseed oil
- 20 drops lemon essential oil

MAKES & KEEPS

Makes ½ cup.
Keeps for years.

METHOD

Heat together the beeswax, turpentine, and linseed oil until the wax melts, being careful not to put it on too high a flame or it will catch fire. Add the lemon essential oil, then pour it into cans while still liquid.

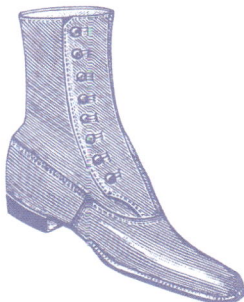

Walnut Protection Remedy

Courtesy of Lucy Harmer

*Helps to relieve the stress of moving and to protect
if you feel unsettled or under attack.*

INGREDIENTS
- **15 green walnuts, cut into 6–8 pieces**
- **2 cups brandy**

MAKES & KEEPS
Makes 2 cups.
Keeps for years.

METHOD
Macerate the walnuts in the brandy for 6 weeks
in a dark place. Stir every 6 days. Strain and
bottle as for tinctures (pp.18–19).

To use, fill a small dropper bottle halfway with
the remedy and top it up with spring water.
Take 3–5 drops 3 times daily whenever you
feel vulnerable.

Sage Smudge Stick

Courtesy of Lucy Harmer

*Smudging, which originates in Native American
traditions, is a great way to cleanse a space, home, or
office. Most smudge sticks are made of sage because
it is such a great purifier.*

INGREDIENTS
- **several small stems fresh sage,
  about 6–15 inches long**

YOU WILL NEED
- THIN STRING OR COTTON YARN ABOUT
  5 FEET LONG

MAKES & KEEPS
Makes 1 stick.
Keeps 1–2 years.

METHOD
Lay the sage stems together so that all the cut
ends are on the same side.

Wind the string or cotton tightly around the
stems, leaving 2 inches of loose string or cotton
where you began. Next, wind the string along
the length of the bundle until you reach the
leafy end. Return to the stem end, thus creating
a crisscross pattern.

When you get back to the stems, tie the
remainder of the string or cotton to the 2-inch
loose piece you left at the beginning.

Hang the bundle up to dry in a dry place
for 3–7 days.

When your smudge stick has dried, you can
light the leafy end. Let it smolder and send
the smoke around a person, an object, or your
home to cleanse and purify. Snuff the sage out
by pressing the stick down on a plate or small
bowl—do not extinguish with water, because it
is then really difficult to light again.

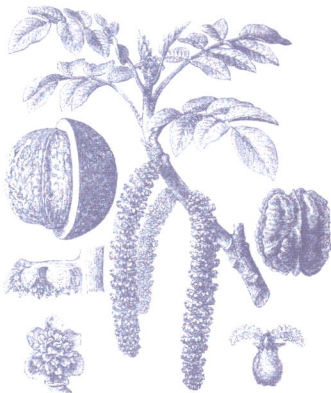

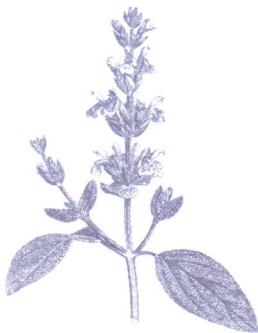

Sage & Lavender Smudge Stick

Courtesy of Lucy Harmer

Use to increase mental energy and feel uplifted.

INGREDIENTS
- **5 stems fresh sage, about 6–15 inches long**
- **5 stems fresh sage, about 6–8 inches long**
- **5 stems fresh lavender, about 6–8 inches long**

YOU WILL NEED
· THIN STRING OR COTTON YARN ABOUT 5 FEET LONG

MAKES & KEEPS
Makes 1 stick.
Keeps 1–2 years.

METHOD
Make as for the Sage Smudge Stick (opposite).

— *Variation* —

ADD A LITTLE FRESH MUGWORT TO THIS BUNDLE FOR A MORE HEALING VIBRATION.

Protection Smudge Stick

Courtesy of Lucy Harmer

Use to clear out and cleanse a space from all negative energy and outside influences.

INGREDIENTS
- **3 stems fresh rosemary, about 6–15 inches long**
- **3 stems fresh lavender, about 6–15 inches long**
- **3 stems fresh juniper, about 6–15 inches long**

YOU WILL NEED
· THIN STRING OR COTTON YARN ABOUT 5 FEET LONG

MAKES & KEEPS
Makes 1 stick.
Keeps 1–2 years.

METHOD
Make as for the Sage Smudge Stick (opposite).

Herbal House Cleansing Stick

Courtesy of Lucy Harmer

An ancient European technique for clearing domestic space.

INGREDIENTS
- **2 cups spring water**
- **3 large pinches of salt**
- **2 sprigs fresh mint**
- **2 sprigs fresh rosemary**
- **2 sprigs fresh marjoram**

MAKES & KEEPS
Makes enough for 1 use.
Use immediately.

METHOD
Pour the water into a bowl and add the salt.

Weave the herb sprigs together to make a thick loose stick.

Dip the stick in the salt water. Sprinkle around the inside and outside of the home.

Happy Home Charm

Courtesy of Lucy Harmer

A traditional European charm.

INGREDIENTS
- pinch of dried rue
- 2 oak leaves
- 3 dead bumblebees
  (that have died naturally)

YOU WILL NEED
· A SMALL POUCH OF NATURAL CLOTH

MAKES & KEEPS
Makes 1 charm.
Keeps 1 year.

METHOD
Put the ingredients into the pouch, thinking of your goal. Hang the pouch next to the front door.

House Protection Charm

Courtesy of Lucy Harmer

INGREDIENTS
- 1 tsp. dried vervain
- 1 tsp. dill seeds
- 1 tsp. dried rosemary leaves
- 1 tsp. dried bay leaves
- 1 tsp. dried St. John's wort
- 1 tsp. juniper berries
- pinch of salt

YOU WILL NEED
· A SMALL POUCH OF NATURAL CLOTH

MAKES & KEEPS
Makes 1 charm.
Keeps 1 year.

METHOD
Put the ingredients into the pouch, thinking of your goal.

Squeeze the pouch to release the herbs' fragrance. Hang next to the front door to bring protection to your home and ward off evil.

Good Sleep Charm

Courtesy of Lucy Harmer

INGREDIENTS
- 2 tsp. dried mugwort
- 2 tsp. dried rue
- 2 tsp. dried lavender
- 2 tsp. dried angelica
- 2 tsp. dried chamomile

YOU WILL NEED
· A SMALL POUCH OF NATURAL CLOTH

MAKES & KEEPS
Makes 1 charm.
Keeps 1 year.

METHOD
Put the ingredients into the pouch, thinking of your goal.

Squeeze the pouch to release the herbs' fragrance. Hang on a bedpost or place under your pillow for protection while asleep and for good dreams.

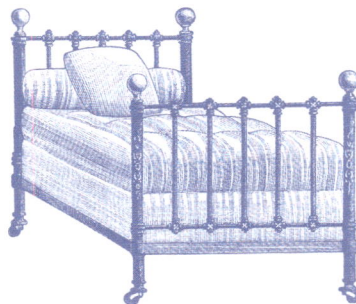

Good Luck Charm

Courtesy of Lucy Harmer

INGREDIENTS
- 4 oak leaves
- small piece of dried heather
- I tsp. dried orange peel
- I acorn
- I citrine quartz crystal

YOU WILL NEED
- A SMALL POUCH OF NATURAL CLOTH

MAKES & KEEPS
Makes I charm.
Keeps I year.

METHOD
Put the ingredients into the pouch, thinking of your goal.

Squeeze the pouch to release the herbs' fragrance. Hang it next to the front door or carry it with you through the day.

Prosperous House Charm

Courtesy of Lucy Harmer

INGREDIENTS
- I tsp. oats
- I tsp. cloves
- I tsp. small pieces of cinnamon stick
- I tsp. mandrake root
- few gold flakes

YOU WILL NEED
- A SMALL POUCH OF NATURAL CLOTH

MAKES & KEEPS
Makes I charm.
Keeps I year.

METHOD
Put the ingredients into the pouch, thinking of your goal.

Squeeze the pouch to release the herbs' fragrance. Hang it next to the front door to bring abundance and wealth to your home.

Herbal Mouse Deterrent

INGREDIENTS
- I cup water
- 2 tbsp. basil
- 2 tbsp. peppermint

Essential oils:
- 2 tsp. peppermint
- 2 tsp. rosemary
- 2 tsp. clove

MAKES & KEEPS
Makes I cup.
Keeps 6 months.

METHOD
Pour boiling water on the herbs and let cool. Strain and add the essential oils to the strong herb tea liquid. Mix well.

Soak a cotton ball thoroughly in the strong-smelling mix. Place around the mouse's entry point to your home. Repeat every 2–4 weeks.

Stinging Nettle String

INGREDIENTS

- 10 or more fresh nettle stems (tall, long straight ones are needed)

MAKES & KEEPS
Keeps indefinitely.

METHOD
Wearing gloves, pull the nettle out of the ground. Rub the stinging hairs and strip the leaves off the stem.

Cut about 1 inch off the bottom and top pieces of the stem.

Crush the stem all along with your fingers. Put a fingernail in at the bottom and open it up all the way along to the top, spreading it open like a book.

Bend the flattened stem over a finger, with the inside facing upward to snap the inside fibers. Carefully peel off and discard these.

The nettle's tough outside fibers can be braided to make a cord. Take 2 or more fibers together and secure one end. Twist both from the other end, then fold them in half. The 2 twisted sides will twist together and naturally form a strong cord.

Let the cord dry somewhere warm for 2 hours.

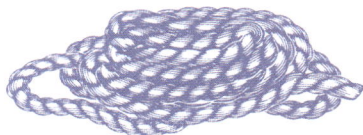

Pungent Pest Control Spray for Plants

Controls pests on outdoor or indoor plants without harming the plant.

INGREDIENTS

- 6 large fresh chiles
- 2 cups water
- 1 head garlic, peeled and crushed

MAKES & KEEPS
Makes nearly 2 cups.
Keeps about 1 week in the refrigerator.

METHOD
Boil the chiles in the water for 15 minutes. Add the garlic and let steep for several hours or overnight. Strain well through cheesecloth and put in a spray bottle ready to use.

Spray affected plants thoroughly, coating the leaves, stems, and soil.

Caution

Best used outside. Be careful when spraying because the chile can really sting if it gets up your nose or in your eyes. Keep away from children or pets.

Tobacco & Tea Tree Plant Spray

An effective remedy against many insects.

INGREDIENTS
- **2 cups boiling water**
- **I handful of tobacco (such as a cheap pipe tobacco)**
- **I00 drops/I tsp. tea tree essential oil**

MAKES & KEEPS
Makes nearly 2 cups.
Keeps about 5 days in the refrigerator.

METHOD
Pour the boiling water over the tobacco. Let cool. Strain and add the tea tree essential oil and put in a spray bottle.

Spray affected plants.

Eco-Sudsy Car Soap

A soapy mix that is perfect for washing the car.

INGREDIENTS
- **I cup liquid soap**
- **¼ cup laundry powder**
- **I large pail of water**

MAKES & KEEPS
Makes I wash.

METHOD
Mix the ingredients together as you need them.

Wash the car with the mixture. Rinse well, then use Plant Power Car Wax (right).

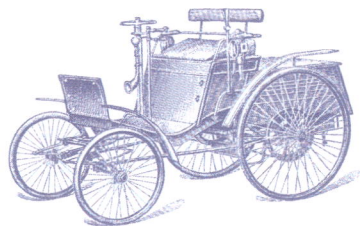

Plant Power Car Wax

This lemony wax uses carnauba—a rich, thick wax from the leaves of the carnauba palm from Brazil. You can make this without the carnauba if you can't get it, but it won't be as long-lasting or effective.

INGREDIENTS
- **I cup linseed oil**
- **¼ cup carnauba wax**
- **2 tbsp. beeswax**
- **I½ cups infused lemon vinegar (p.I9)**

MAKES & KEEPS
Makes about 3 cups.
Keeps indefinitely.

METHOD
Heat the ingredients gently (in a double boiler) until the wax has melted. Stir, then pour into a heat-resistant container.

When the mixture is cool, it will solidify. Rub it on the car with a lint-free cloth. Polish to a deep shine with the corner of a cotton duster soaked in vinegar.

Herb Directory

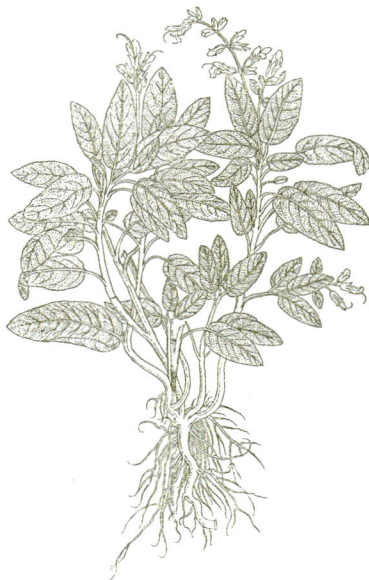

ACHILLEA MILLEFOLIUM
Yarrow

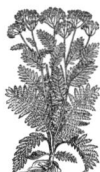

Long used to staunch wounds (on battlefields and elsewhere), yarrow's pinky white flowers and feathery leaves grace many a field and grassland area in temperate zones across the world.

USES *Yarrow is used to treat period pains, high blood pressure, blood vessel problems, fevers, and respiratory allergies; it can also improve digestion. Although yarrow stops hemorrhaging, taken both internally and used externally, the leaves and flowers are anticlotting for the circulatory system. Take as tea, tincture, lotion, salve, or poultice.*

Its root secretions are known to be strengthening to other plants, making them more resistant to disease, and the plant repels harmful insects in the yard.

Some people are allergic to yarrow. Do not use in pregnancy.

AGRIMONIA SSP.
Agrimony

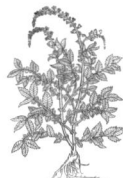

A 3-foot tall perennial herb with carrotlike leaves, agrimony is green on top and silvery underneath, with thin spikes of small yellow flowers. It prefers a wet habitat.

USES *Agrimony's main quality is its astringency, which means it is drying and toning to mucous membranes. This makes it useful to tone the digestive system, and as a mouthwash for gum disease. It is used to treat bladder and kidney weakness.*

Agrimony is also a flower remedy for tension and pressure, especially for those who put on a brave face. Externally, it is an excellent healer of wounds, including varicose ulcers. Take as a tea, tincture, or external preparation.

AESCULUS HIPPOCASTANUM
Horse Chestnut

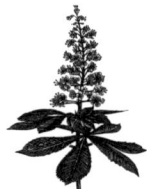

This majestic tree, a native of southeastern Europe, is now cultivated throughout the world. It produces fragrant candles of small flowers and a profusion of brown, shiny, nutlike seeds, protected by spiky green cases.

USES *The seeds, or "conkers," are used in internal and external medicines to strengthen blood vessels, especially the veins. In large doses, horse chestnuts are poisonous— do not mistake it for sweet chestnut and eat too many.*

The safe medicinal dose is about 1–2g three times daily. Take as a tincture or in powder form, or apply as a lotion or cream.

ALCHEMILLA VULGARIS
Lady's Mantle

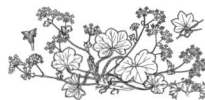

This delicate, yellow-green plant has soft, capelike leaves that collect dew and tiny, green-yellow flowers. It is usually found in damp meadows, woods, and grassy mountains.

USES *An excellent general tonic for the womb, lady's mantle stops excess bleeding—menstrual or menopausal— and regulates the female hormonal cycle. The herb also helps women to recover from emotional and physical trauma related to the womb. Being astringent, it can ease diarrhea and mucous problems of the digestive tract. Its astringency, coupled with an ability to stem bleeding, makes lady's mantle a good healer of wounds. Take as a tea or a tincture, or in a healing salve or poultice. It is not generally used in pregnancy.*

ALLIUM SATIVUM
Garlic

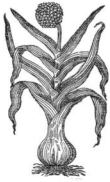

The bulb of this typical, easy to grow member of the onion family is used in cooking all over the world. Its cousin, *Allium ursinum* (wild garlic, bear garlic, or ramsons)—available online to grow from seeds—grows all over Europe and can be used similarly.

USES *Garlic is highly effective in fighting infections of all kinds, including coughs and colds, sinusitis, and intestinal parasites. Used in treating hay fever and other allergies, it can also lower blood cholesterol and high blood pressure.*

Some research has found it to be a possible neurotoxin that adversely affects the brain, so it may be best regarded as a medicine for occasional use. Garlic can be eaten raw or made into a powerful tincture, or applied externally to infections.

ALTHAEA OFFICINALIS
Marshmallow

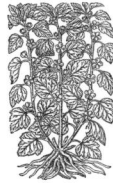

Originally from Africa and now widely cultivated, marshmallow is a tall perennial herb. It has pale pink flowers and soft, furry, light green leaves.

USES *The leaves and root are used to soften and soothe inflammations of the lungs, digestive tract, urinary tract, and skin. The root tends to be used more for digestion and lungs, the leaves for the kidneys.*

The root can be chewed by teething babies. In ancient Egypt, marshmallow was mixed with oats and honey to make a sacred confectionery offered to the gods.

ALOE VERA
Aloe

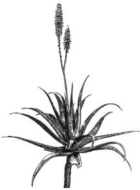

This cactuslike plant has long, pointed, succulent leaves edged with small white teeth. It is good to grow as a houseplant, so you can split the dark green leaves, reach the clear gel within, and use it fresh.

USES *Aloe juice is rich in vitamins, minerals, and health-giving enzymes. It is powerfully detoxifying and an excellent cleanser. Anti-inflammatory for the stomach and colon, aloe juice is used to treat irritable bowel syndrome (IBS) and other digestive inflammations. It helps to heal burns and ulcers and is used in many skin products.*

Do not take in pregnancy or when breastfeeding, or if the kidneys are weak. Do not take internally long-term without regular breaks.

ANGELICA ARCHANGELICA
Angelica

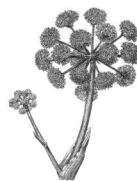

A tall and powerful aromatic bitter of the Umbelliferae family, angelica has tiny flowers with distinctive, umbrella-shape flower heads. Angelica is found most often growing alongside rivers, preferring damp and shady places. Originally native to Syria, it is now widely cultivated.

Be careful when collecting this herb because angelica can easily be mistaken for hemlock, which is poisonous.

USES *Stems and roots can be eaten. In medicinal terms, angelica is an aromatic bitter that removes damp and cold from the body. It stimulates the liver and digestive tracts, and is a valuable tonic for the whole system. The root is especially useful for the lungs. All parts of the plant are used, in teas, tinctures, and foods. Do not take medicinally during pregnancy.*

ARCTIUM LAPPA
Burdock

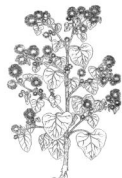

In burdock's first year, only the leaves appear. They are low to the ground, large, and flannelly, with a distinctive smell and feel, being woolly on the underside. In its second year, the plant grows a tall, robust stem with leaves and small pinky purple, thistlelike flowers, which form seed burrs. Native to Europe, it is naturalized in the United States.

USES *Burdock is a blood-cleansing herb that is antibiotic, antifungal, and adaptagenic (protects the body from stress). It lowers blood sugar, stimulates the kidneys, promotes sweating, and is used to treat many skin diseases, as well as arthritis and any condition where detoxifying is necessary. The root, leaves, and seeds are used in teas, tinctures, and foods.*

ARMORACIA RUSTICANA
Horseradish

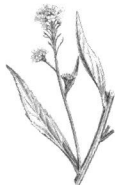

Horseradish is a member of the cabbage family native to Europe and western Asia, then introduced to North America. It has strong, large green leaves and small white flowers.

USES *Though best known as a culinary herb, horseradish root is a useful antibiotic and immune-stimulating medicine. It is especially good for infections of the sinuses, lungs, kidneys, and digestive tract, and removal of mucus from the body. It is also a strong diuretic that breaks up kidney stones and a stimulant for the circulation.*

Horseradish is easy to grow and best used fresh. It is taken internally as a tincture, tea, and food, and used externally in lotions.

ARTEMISIA ABSINTHIUM
Wormwood

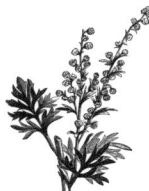

This bitter herb with small yellow flowers is native to Europe, but now also grown in Asia and the United States. It can easily be grown from seed or by dividing the roots in fall.

USES *Wormwood is used to treat parasite infections of the digestive tract and as a general tonic. It is a bitter liver stimulant that affects the central nervous system, and is best used in small amounts. Wormwood was a key ingredient in the liquor "absinthe," which has mind-altering effects.*

Its cousin, A. annua, or Chinese wormwood, has been found to be effective against malaria. In countries where the disease is prevalent, there have been programs to encourage growing of Chinese wormwood for use in treatments.

Do not take during pregnancy.

ARTEMISIA VULGARIS
Mugwort

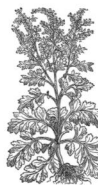

Also known as Chrysanthamum weed, mugwort grows over most of Europe and North America. The under leaves are white, the flowers white-green and small, but they grow in profuse spikes.

USES *Mugwort leaves and flower buds can be used to flavor soups or eaten for their minerals (and their ability to help the body absorb minerals). It is a bitter liver tonic of particular help to the womb, nervous system, and stomach.*

Mugwort can be taken as a tea or tincture, and can be smoked, like a cigarette, or burned as an incense. It is also used in acupuncture in a procedure called "moxibustion," where it is burned into the patient's skin. Mugwort is said to help to develop lucid (conscious) dreaming.

Do not take during pregnancy.

ASTRAGALUS MEMBRANACEUS
Huang Qi or Milk Vetch

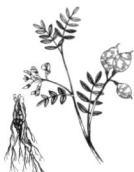

The root of this yellow-flowered member of the vetch family has been used for thousands of years in Chinese medicine for its invigorating qualities. It is native to temperate regions of the Northern Hemisphere.

USES *A tonic for the immune system, milk vetch increases our ability to fight off viral disease. It supports the immune system, so helps with chronic fatigue, and also supports people having chemotherapy and radiation therapy. Milk vetch is a general tonic for the digestion, heart, and liver, and may also be used to help prolapsed organs, especially the womb. The root is decocted into a tea or made into a tincture.*

BAPTISIA TINCTORIA
Horseflyweed/Wild Indigo

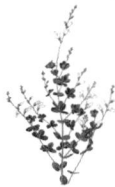

A yellow-flowered perennial in the vetch family, horseflyweed is native to North America. Widely used in herbal medicine, where it is also known as wild indigo, which refers to its traditional use as a blue dye.

USES *Wild indigo root is used in herbal medicine as an antiseptic blood cleanser and to stimulate immunity against infection. It is especially suited for digestive infections, including typhus, gastric flu, mouth infections, and sepsis anywhere in the body.*

AVENA SATIVA
Oat Straw

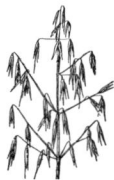

Oats are a tall grass with straight stems and small seed heads. Herbalists use "oat straw"—the green grass and tops of oats before the mature oats are formed—as a powerful medicine. It is native to temperate parts of Europe and Asia, and is widely cultivated around the world.

USES *Superrich in minerals and vitamins, oats are a nutritious, health-enhancing, cholesterol-lowering food.*

A tonic and nourishing herb for the nerves, including the brain, oat straw is used for fatigue, depression, and anxiety, and to improve concentration. It can help with insomnia caused by overexhaustion and may also be used as an aphrodisiac and reproductive tonic. It is taken as a tea or tincture; the grass may be eaten in green smoothies.

BERBERIS VULGARIS
Barberry

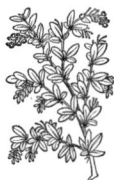

Barberry is a thorny deciduous shrub from Africa, Asia, and southern Europe, now naturalized in the United States. It has small, leathery leaves, yellow bark, and flowers and red berries.

USES *In many countries, barberry's tart red berries are eaten in savory dishes and preserves. The yellow bark of its stem and root are used as a dye and a powerful medicine.*

Barberry contains berberine, an antibacterial, antiprotozoal, and antiparasite antibiotic that is also anti-inflammatory. Used for intestinal infections and eye infections, parasites, and malaria, barberry is a bitter stimulant for the liver.

Do not take during pregnancy or long-term (more than 2 months).

MAHONIA AQUIFOLIUM
Oregon Grape

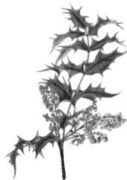

Also known as hollyleaved barberry, Oregon grape is an evergreen from North America in the Berberidaceae family, now grown in Europe. Growing to 6 feet, it has prickly, hollylike leaves, clusters of yellow flowers, and small black berries.

USES *A bitter tonic for the liver and digestive system, Oregon grape also contains berberine (so can be used in a similar way to barberry, p. 227). It is much used to treat psoriasis, eczema, and other skin diseases, being a detoxifier and tonic.*

The inner bark produces a yellow dye, the berries a purple one. Berries can also be eaten, usually cooked and mixed with a sweeter fruit. The root is used in medicines.

Do not take during pregnancy.

CALENDULA OFFICINALIS
Pot Marigold

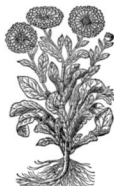

Originally from southern Europe, pot marigold grows in any temperate climate and is now found all over the world. It is easy to grow and ideal for novice gardeners. The vibrant orange flowers have medicinal use.

USES *Pot marigold is one of the most versatile and amazing plants. The anti-inflammatory flowers heal wounds and work against bacteria, viruses, and fungal infections. They are used in preparations for skin problems of all kinds.*

Pot marigold flowers are also effective as a healing remedy for the digestive tract, and for strengthening the liver as well as the nervous system.

BORAGO OFFICINALIS
Borage

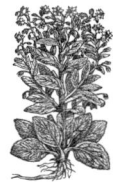

Native to the Mediterranean and widely grown elsewhere, borage is a bristly haired, bright green herb with characteristic blue, star-shape flowers. Star-flower oil is extracted from its seeds. Star-flower oil contains high levels of GLA (gamma linoleic acid), which has many beneficial health effects, including helping to regulate hormone levels, so it can help reduce PMS.

USES *Borage is cooling and moistening, and is used in herbal medicine as an adrenal tonic for stress, exhaustion, and depression. It soothes stomach inflammations and reduces catarrh in the body.*

Borage leaves and flowers can be eaten and are delicious. The leaves contain low levels of pyrrolixidine alkaloids, so there are some concerns about borage's safety, because in high doses these damage the liver. Take borage for only a few weeks at a time, and do not take if you have any liver disease or weakness. If in doubt, consult a medical herbalist.

CAPSICUM SPP.
Cayenne Pepper

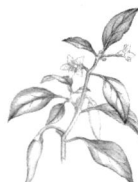

Cayenne is a hot chile pepper with long green "fruits," which usually turn red on ripening. It is native to both South and Central America.

USES *Cayenne pepper fruits are taken as a powerful circulatory stimulant, dilating blood vessels and speeding up flow around the body. The plant speeds up metabolism, helps to burn fat, and suppresses the appetite: it is also said to be an aphrodisiac.*

Cayenne pepper is consumed as a powder or tincture, or taken externally as a warming pain-killer. It is also used as a spray to deter insects on other plants. Do not use on broken skin or delicate areas, and keep away from the eyes.

Do not take medicinal doses in pregnancy.

CHELIDONIUM MAJUS
Greater Celandine

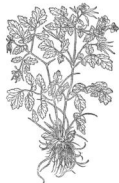

A member of the poppy family with small yellow flowers, the stem of greater celandines produces an orange latex. (Latex is a milky exudate that some plants contain, including opium in poppies and rubber from rubber plants.) Native to Europe, it is widely grown in the United States.

USES   *A bitter tonic for all manner of liver and gall-bladder diseases, greater celandine is also a mild sedative for the internal organs. It is used to treat whooping cough, asthma and bronchitis with spasm, and for pain in the digestive system. The herb is taken and applied for eczema, and for eye disease and cancers. It is used as a tea, tincture and lotion, and the latex can be directly applied to warts.*

Do not take during pregnancy.

CRATAEGUS MONOGYNA
Hawthorn

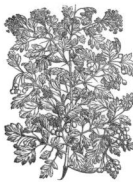

This wonderful common hedge plant and field tree with its rugged bark, profusion of white-pink flowers, and red berries is found throughout Europe. Several North American cousins have similar medicinal properties, including *Crataegus chrysocarpa* (fireberry hawthorn) and *C. douglasii* (black hawthorn) as well as *C. pinnatifida* (Chinese hawthorn).

USES   *In German herbal medicine, hawthorn is known as "the mother of the heart," and its flowering tops and berries are used to treat all manner of heart disease: angina, abnormal heart rhythms, heart failure, high blood pressure, and diseases of the arteries.*

CIMICIFUGA RACEMOSA
Black Cohosh

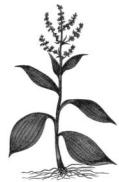

A graceful woodland perennial native to the United States and now naturalized in Europe, black cohosh has long, bending spikes of white flowers (3 feet in length). Now reclassified as *Actaea racemosa* and sometimes called black baneberry, black cohosh root was traditionally used for medicine by many Native American tribes.

USES   *An anti-inflammatory, black cohosh is helpful for sciatica, back pain, cramp, arthritis, and is sometimes used for migraines. It is a relaxing nerve tonic that can quieten a cough.*

Black cohosh can also be helpful for period pains, and for painful breasts and headaches caused by hormonal imbalance, as well as menopausal hot sweats.

Do not use in pregnancy or when breastfeeding. Do not take for more than 6 months without a break.

CURCUMA LONGA
Turmeric

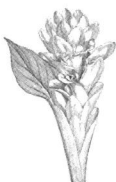

This tropical plant is native to South India, and is widely grown in hot and wet areas of the tropics. Its large green leaves grow to around 3 feet and its flowers are whitish green. The yellow rhizomes (roots) are used in cooking. Turmeric is considered to be an exceptionally powerful medicinal plant.

USES   *A supreme anti-inflammatory, liver activator, and antioxidant blood cleanser, turmeric is useful in any inflammatory condition. These include arthritis, skin disorders, asthma, cancers, and heart disease. The herb has been shown to be of help in dementia and diabetes. It is normally used in dried powder form because it is imported from India, but if you can get turmeric fresh, try eating it grated, or as a juice—it is amazing. It also makes a bold yellow dye.*

229

DIOSCOREA VILLOSA
Wild Yam

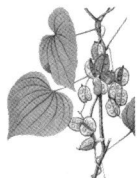

Native to North and Central America, wild yam will grow in subtropical and temperate zone woodlands. It consists of a vine growing from tubers (potato-like roots), which are the part used in medicine.

USES *Wild yam is traditionally used as an anti-spasmodic, especially for digestive tract spasm or colic, and also as an anti-inflammatory for inflamed bowels and arthritic conditions. It is also used to treat women's hormonal imbalances; common in menopausal mixes, the plant is famous for containing diosgenin, from which the first contraceptive pill was developed. It is taken as a tea, tincture, and cream.*

ELEUTHEROCOCCUS SENTICOSUS
Siberian Ginseng

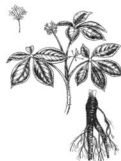

Native to Russia, China, Korea, and Japan, Siberian ginseng is a woody shrub, 10 feet in height, with blackish berries and large, dark green leaves with 3–7 lobes.

USES *The root is used as a strong adaptogen (meaning that it helps protect the body from the damaging effects of stress) and stimulant. It is often used to boost long-term immunity, including for people with immunosuppression following radiation therapy or chemotherapy. Siberian ginseng is helpful in any stress-related condition, including those caused by hormonal problems, such as postnatal depression and menopausal difficulties.*

It is best used for short periods of time. For some people, it is too stimulating, causing anxiety and panic, especially in high doses. Siberian ginseng is mostly used as a tea and tincture.

ECHINACEA SPP. (E. PURPUREA AND E. ANGUSTIFOLIA)
Purple Coneflower

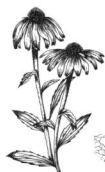

Native to the United States but now cultivated and known far and wide, this perennial boasts a lovely, large, daisy-type purple flower. The whole plant (root and flowering tops) is used for medicine.

USES *Echinacea is an immune stimulant, helping the body to fight infections and cleaning the blood. It is antimicrobial and can be used to treat boils, ulcers, eczema, and any infection anywhere in the body. Good-quality echinacea makes the tongue tingle when you taste it or chew it. It is taken as a tincture, tea, and pills.*

EQUISETUM SPP. (E.ARVENSE AND E. HYEMALE)
Horsetail

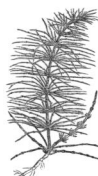

This ancient plant with thin, rigid, dry branching stems and leaves resembles a horse's tail. It likes wet, marshy places and grows up to 2 feet in height.

USES *Horsetail is rich in silica in a readily absorbable form. A lack of silica can be recognized by weakness of the hair and nails, multiple allergies, chronic bladder inflammation, and muscle and joint problems.*

Horsetail helps to stop bleeding, especially of the bladder and reproductive organs, and is also used for urinary incontinence.

Be careful not to confuse it with E. palustre *(marsh horsetail), which is much larger and is toxic.*

FILIPENDULA ULMARIA
Meadowsweet

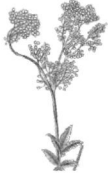

Also known as Queen of the Meadow, this lovely herbaceous perennial, with its shower of creamy-white flowers and distinctive smell, is native to Europe and Asia and naturalized in the United States.

USES *Meadowsweet is a useful anti-inflammatory for the stomach and intestines, and for the joints. It relieves and heals stomach ulcers and heartburn and calms an overactive digestion, so can help to stop diarrhea. The herb also contains salicylic acid (aspirin), so lowers fevers and thins blood.*

GENTIANA LUTEA
Gentian

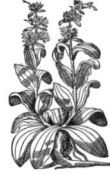

Gentian grows in the Alps and other mountainous regions. It has oval leaves and star-shape yellow flowers, and grows to around 4 feet in height. Its bitter roots are collected in fall from plants that are more than 8 years old, which is when they first begin to flower.

USES *Gentian stimulates the liver and digestion, regulates blood sugar, and is a general tonic. It is used usually in small quantities, with a tincture of the root normally being taken at 2—10 drops per dose. Taken directly on the tongue, gentian can help reduce sugar cravings. Avoid if you experience acid indigestion or a stomach ulcer.*

GALIUM APARINE
Cleavers, Goosegrass

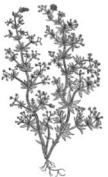

This creeping plant grows all over Europe, North America, and parts of Asia. Cleavers stays close to the ground and climbs over other plants. Its hairy stems are square, its flowers tiny and white, and its fruits resemble little balls.

USES *Cleavers is used to encourage the lymphatic system to detoxify the body. It is taken for any condition in which toxic buildup could be an issue, including conditions of the skin and joints and certain cancers.*

GINKGO BILOBA
Ginkgo

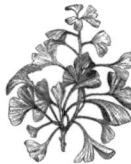

This magnificent and ancient tree, with green, fan-shape leaves, has been around for about 190 million years. Growing to 100 feet, it is native to China and Japan, but is now grown all over the world.

USES *The leaves are famous as a brain medicine, stimulating the flow of blood to the brain. Ginkgo is used to treat memory loss and problems of the central nervous system, including dementia, stroke, and multiple sclerosis. It has an anticlotting effect in the blood.*

Ginkgo can also help with asthma, being strongly anti-allergic and anti-inflammatory. It is usually taken in tincture or pill form, or as powder.

GLYCYRRHIZA GLABRA
Licorice

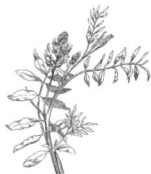

A woody stemmed member of the pea family, with creamy-white flowers, licorice is native to southern Europe and Asia. It is now widely cultivated.

USES *Licorice is famous as a confectionery, full of delicious natural sugars. It is such a useful medicine that it has been called "the universal herb."*

An adrenal tonic for exhaustion and fatigue, it is anti-inflammatory for the stomach and digestive tract and soothes the lungs and urinary system. Licorice also heals externally and can help ulcers and eczema (it makes an especially black ointment).

Do not use during pregnancy, or with liver damage or high blood pressure.

INULA HELENIUM
Elecampane

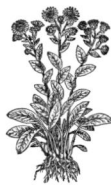

This robust member of the daisy family is native to Europe, but naturalized in the United States. It grows in many places, preferring shady woods and damp pastures. It grows 3–5 feet tall, with yellow flowers and pointed leaves. The root, dug in fall from plants over 2–3 years old, is used for medicine.

USES *Elecampane root is a warming tonic, especially good for the lungs; it treats coughs, catarrh, and serious lung disorders of all kinds. Elecampane root is also useful to improve digestion and to treat hemorrhoids, debility, and exhaustion.*

Do not take during pregnancy or if breastfeeding.

HYPERICUM PERFORATUM
St. John's Wort

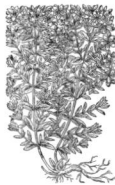

This beautiful wayside weed with small yellow flowers is indigenous to Europe, but introduced in temporate zones of the Americas. If you hold the leaves up to the light, you will find little see-through dots; these are oil glands.

USES *In addition to its now famous use as an antidepressant, St. John's wort is taken as a tea, capsules, or tincture for stress and anxiety, and to treat damage to and diseases of the nerves (including shingles and multiple sclerosis). It supports the immune system and stimulates the liver. The lovely infused oil is anti-inflammatory, antiviral, and wound-healing.*

It can cause sensitivity to sunlight and interacts with some medicines, including the oral contraceptive pill. Seek medical advice if you are taking any medication.

IRIS VERSICOLOR
Blue Flag

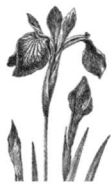

This beautiful wetland iris, a native of North America, has characteristic purple yellow and whitish flowers much loved by florists. The root is used in herbal medicine throughout the USA and Europe.

USES *Used in small doses, the root has the action of stimulating a sluggish liver; it also improves eczema and other skin diseases, encourages the lymphatic system, and moves the bowels. Blue flag root is useful for acne, psoriasis, and shingles, and can also help people with an underactive thyroid.*

Do not take in pregnancy. It can also cause vomiting in large doses.

JUGLANS NIGRA
Black Walnut

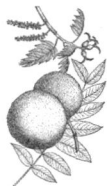

This beautiful tree is native to the United States but has been widely introduced in Europe. It produces a fruit that falls with its husk, green, in fall, and this green fruit, as well as the leaves and flowers, all have medicinal uses.

USES *The nuts are delicious and nutritious. Interestingly, they are especially good for the brain—they even look like little brains!*

Black walnut calms inflammation of the bowels and parasite infestation. It also improves digestion and cleans the blood.

Walnut hulls make a brownish black dye, while the flower makes a remedy to help adjust to periods of change.

Do not use walnut hulls during pregnancy; the flower remedy is fine at this time.

LARREA TRIDENTATA
Creosote Bush

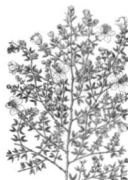

This fragrant evergreen shrub is a familiar sight in the deserts of the southwestern United States and northwestern Mexico. Growing to 3–9 feet in height, it has dark green leaves and yellow flowers.

USES *Tea made from creosote leaves was traditionally used for detoxification, and to treat colds and pain from kidney stones.*

Creosote bush is antifungal, antimicrobial, antiviral, and anti-inflammatory; it is also astringent and antioxidant. The plant makes a wonderful infused oil that heals wounds and soothes inflammations, bruises, and skin infections when applied to the skin.

It may be harmful to the liver taken in large doses over a long period, or in susceptible individuals, so do not take it internally unless done under the guidance of a qualified herbalist.

LACTUCA SPP.
Wild Lettuce

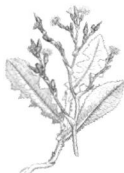

The wild cousin of all the cultivated varieties, wild lettuce has small, slightly prickly leaves and yellow flowers. It is much more bitter than cultivated lettuce. Native to Asia and Europe, it is naturalized in the United States.

USES *Remember* The Tale of Peter Rabbit? *He ate too many of Mr. McGregor's lettuces and fell asleep ... Wild lettuce has a latex (a white waxy juice that oozes from the fresh stems), which contains an opiate. The latex forms an opiate-like sedative and pain-killer used to treat insomnia, hyperactivity, anxiety, and pain of various kinds.*

Wild lettuce is taken in herbal medicine as a tea or tincture. In large doses it causes drowsiness.

LAVANDULA ANGUSTIFOLIA AND SPP.
Lavender

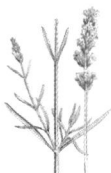

This aromatic, purple-flowered perennial prefers dry, well drained soil and plenty of sun. It is grown commercially mainly for production of its essential oil, which is antiseptic and anti-inflammatory. Many related species have similar properties. It has been cultivated across Europe, Asia, and Africa for thousands of years.

USES *Lavender is used in cooking cakes and desserts, and sometimes for flavoring cheese.*

Medicinally, the herb is relaxing and antiseptic. It encourages liver function and is used to treat high blood pressure, exhaustion, anxiety, insomnia, headaches, and painful spasms.

The oil is used neat to heal burns and wounds, and is often used in household and personal care products. It is used also as a tea, tincture, and aromatic water. Do not take essential oils internally without professional supervision.

233

LEONURUS CARDIACA
Motherwort

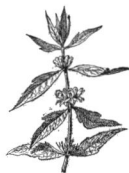

Originally from southern Europe and Asia, motherwort long ago spread across the world. This tall, strong perennial of the mint family has hairy, serrated, 3–5-lobed leaves, and lilac to pink flowers around the upper parts of the plant.

USES *From the bitter taste, you can tell that motherwort stimulates the liver (as all bitter herbs do). Its names reflect its main medicinal uses—as an herb to strengthen the heart ("lionheart" in Latin) and to treat women's conditions. Motherwort was particularly used to prevent women developing uterine infections after childbirth, and is still widely taken for menopausal difficulties, especially nervous problems. It is an excellent remedy for heart palpitations and weakness, hence its bold Latin name. It is commonly taken as a tea and tincture.*

MATRICARIA CHAMOMILLA
Chamomile

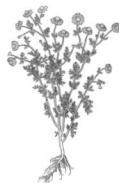

Or German chamomile, a much-loved member of the daisy family with small yellow and white flowers and a distinctive fragrance. It is native to Europe and Asia. A close relative, *Anthemis nobile* or Roman chamomile, is similarly used.

USES *Known as "the mother of the gut," chamomile is a relaxing, antispasmodic sedative. It is used for all inflammations of the digestive tract, from top to bottom, and also helps insomnia.*

Chamomile is a mild emmenegogue, meaning it can bring on delayed menstruation, and it has been used traditionally as a tea to treat vomiting in pregnancy. (Pregnant women should not use the essential oil.)

Used as a tea, tincture, infused oil, or essential oil, chamomile is also soothing for the skin. People allergic to ragwort are sometimes also sensitive to chamomile.

LOBELIA INFLATA
Lobelia

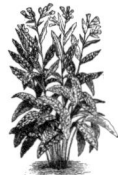

This hairy-stemmed plant has toothed leaves and small, pale purple flowers that are yellowish inside. It is native to the United States.

USES *Lobelia contains strong alkaloids that relax the muscles; it is particularly good for asthma because it will open and relax the respiratory passages. It can be taken internally, and also applied externally, to relieve muscle spasms and cramps.*

If you are giving up smoking, put a drop or two of the tincture directly on your tongue if you need help to reduce cravings.

Treat lobelia with respect because it is strong. It will make you sick in large amounts, so can be used as an emetic.

MELISSA OFFICINALIS
Lemon Balm

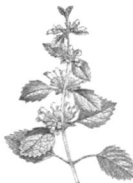

This sweetly lemon-scented hardy perennial is naturalized all over the United States. Similar to mint in appearance, but with bright green leaves and small whitish flowers, it has also been known as "heart's delight."

USES *An effective sedative, lemon balm is good for insomnia, headaches, anxiety, stress, and hyperactivity. The flowering tops are taken to increase mental stamina, and as a digestive herb.*

As well as bringing a fever down, lemon balm is antiviral internally and externally. It is good for cold sores and shingles, and the fresh juice applied to cuts and grazes helps them heal.

Lemon balm is an antihistamine and therefore good for allergies (including eczemas). It is safe for all to take.

MENTHA PIPERITA AND SPP.
Peppermint

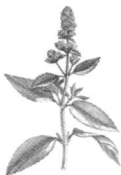

Peppermint is an herbaceous perennial with square stems and opposite dark green pointy leaves, growing 12–35 inches. It is particularly easy to cultivate, spreading by underground roots to form new plants. Mints tend to prefer damp and shady habitats, and are easily recognizable by their distinctive smell and taste.

USES *Rich in an essential oil, which gives it many of its properties, mint gives a sensation of cooling when applied to the skin. It stimulates the liver and digestion, so is useful for nausea and vomiting, indigestion, and heartburn (and often used to treat IBS).*

Mint acts as a stimulant and gives a feeling of improved concentration. It lowers fever, improves appetite, and is a nutritious food. The herb is well used as a tea, oil, and tincture.

ORIGANUM VULGARE
Oregano

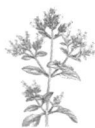

Oregano and its close cousin, *O. marjorana* (marjoram), are native to the Mediterranean and Asia. Both are small-leaved, highly aromatic members of the mint family, with tiny, pink-purple flowers. They prefer the heat and a well-drained soil, but can be surprisingly hardy when grown.

USES *Oregano and marjoram are well-known culinary herbs that lend a distinctive "Italian" flavor to dishes. Both are healthful, nutritious, and tasty additions to the diet. They are used in traditional medicine for their antiseptic properties, especially in treating stomach and respiratory infections. They are aromatic bitters, helping the digestion.*

OCIMUM BASILICUM
Basil

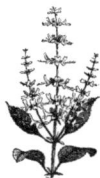

Basil is a strongly aromatic member of the mint family, with shiny green leaves and very small white flowers. Native to India, it has been cultivated in southern Europe and across Asia for thousands of years. It is easy to grow on a sunny windowsill.

USES *Basil is a delicious and versatile culinary herb. An antiviral and antimicrobial plant, it is a superb strengthening tonic for the whole body. It helps the digestion and increases milk flow in nursing mothers. Basil makes a relaxing tonic for the nerves and is good for respiratory ailments.*

Its cousin, O. sanctum, or holy basil, is considered in Ayurvedic medicine to be a supreme healing tonic. It is sacred to Vaisnavas, being Krishna's most beloved plant.

PANAX GINSENG & P. QUINQUEFOLIUS
Chinese Ginseng & American Ginseng

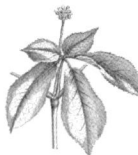

Panax ginseng, a perennial plant in the ivy family, has small red berries and a fleshy root. It is found mainly in Korea and China. American ginseng is similar but native to North America; it is also cultivated in China. They are both particularly prized as medicines.

USES *Ginseng is an "adaptogen," meaning that it protects the body and mind from the damaging effects of stress. It is beneficial to the immune system and can help with recovery from cancer, especially with problems arising from radiation therapy and chemotherapy. It is traditionally used as an aphrodisiac. Too much can lead to agitation (as with too much caffeine).*

PASSIFLORA INCARNATA
Passionflower

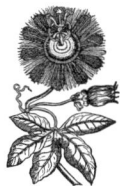

Also known as maypop, this vine has curly tendrils that hang on as it climbs. It produces gorgeous purple flowers, many varieties of which are cultivated for flowers and fruit. It is native to the United States.

USES *The leaves and flowers have long been used as a general relaxing and calming sedative for insomnia and anxiety, epilepsy, and high blood pressure. They are a remedy for twitchy limbs, hyperactivity, pain (in particular nerve pain), and to help manage withdrawal from addictions to alcohol and other drugs.*

Do not take high doses in pregnancy. Passionflower can also cause drowsiness.

PLANTAGO SPP.
Ribwort, Plantain

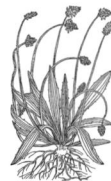

Both herbs are herbaceous perennials. Ribwort (*Plantago lanceolata*), which is also known as narrowleaf plantain, is named for the characteristic veins running straight up the narrow leaves, stem to tip. *Plantago major*, or plantain, is similar, but with round leaves instead of long. The flowers of both are brownish bobbles at the end of long, square stems. They are native to Europe and Asia, and naturalized in the United States.

USES *Plantain/ribwort are so nutritious that the whole body feels their benefit when they are eaten. As a medicine, they tone and dry the mucous membranes of the body, thus helping the lungs, digestive tract, kidney, bladder, and reproductive organs. They help to calm allergies and support the lymphatic system; they are also outstanding wound healers.*

PHYTOLACCA DECANDRA
Poke Root

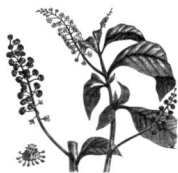

A U.S. native with red stems, narrow green leaves, small, greenish white flowers in spikes, and black berries, pokeroot grows up to 10 feet tall. In large doses it is poisonous, but it is a useful medicine in small amounts.

USES *Poke root helps the lymphatic system and kills parasites in the digestive tract. It is used for sore and swollen glands, for breast disease, and to assist the body to rid itself of cancer.*

The herb is anti-inflammatory when applied externally. A tincture made from the fresh root is used in small amounts, usually not more than 2 tsp. per week (3–4 drops per dose).

Large doses cause vomiting. Do not use in pregnancy.

POLYGONATUM BIFLORUM
Smooth Solomon's Seal

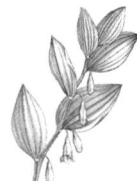

Native to the United States and China, Solomon's seal is cultivated as a garden plant in Europe for its elegant arched stems, from which hang many small white flowers.

USES *The young shoots and leaves can be boiled like asparagus, and the rhizomes ground to make flour for baking.*

The root is taken and applied externally for arthritis and any musculoskeletal problem, including injuries. Additionally it is a soothing demulcent (meaning it has a softening action) for the lungs and digestion and an adrenal tonic that supports the heart, liver, and kidneys. Solomon's seal is a mild sedative and sometimes helps diabetes and high blood pressure.

The aerial parts, especially the berries, are poisonous.

ROSA SPP.
Rose

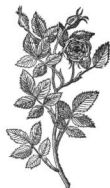

There are more than a hundred species of roses found all over the world. The ones advisable to use for medicine or food include *R. canina*, *R. arkansa*, *R. laevigata*, and *R. rugosa*.

USES *The flowers are edible, as are the fruits; known as "hips," they are exceptionally rich in vitamin C. The seeds contain an oil, which is extracted as an antioxidant and scar-reducing agent. Rose is also known to reduce the effects of aging when applied to the skin.*

Taken internally, rose is an uplifting herb. Helpful to the stomach and digestion, it is also a liver stimulant and tonic for the womb and kidneys. Some species have anticancer activity.

Use the listed wild species for food and medicine, not garden hybrids.

RUBUS IDAEUS
Raspberry

This red-fruited plant with a light green prickly stem and leaves that are green on top and white underneath is native to Europe and Asia, but now widely grown. Its close cousins have similar actions. For example, the U.S. black raspberry is a super antioxidant, which seems to have anticancer benefits.

USES *The fruit is a delicious and healthy food, rich in antioxidants. Leaves can be taken as a womb tonic for threatened miscarriage, to prepare for pregnancy, or as part of infertility treatment. It is also taken as a tea for the last 2–4 months of pregnancy to prepare for childbirth, and taken after birth to nourish the uterus and increase milk production.*

Raspberry's astringency makes it useful to treat diarrhea, and as a wash for canker sores and tonsillitis.

ROSMARINUS OFFICINALIS
Rosemary

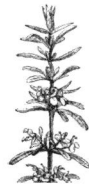

This aromatic, perennial, woody-stemmed shrub is native to the Mediterranean and needs plenty of sunlight to flourish fully. Its green-white, needlelike leaves and purple, pink, white, or blue flowers smell strongly of the essential oil in which rosemary is rich.

USES *Both the fresh and dried herb and the essential oil are often used in medicines, foods, and household products as a good antibacterial.*

Rosemary promotes the circulation, especially the blood flow to the brain. It is used to treat headaches, depression, and weakness, to stimulate the liver and digestion, and to strengthen the heart.

Make a tea or tincture of the flowering tops for internal use. Do not take the essential oil internally without some professional supervision.

SALIX ALBA AND SPP.
White Willow

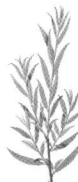

These beautiful trees love damp places, especially riverbanks. They have flexible wood and green-white leaves, and bees love their small, pollen-rich flowers. The anti-inflammatory medicine salicylic acid (aspirin) was first isolated from white willow bark in 1838. Willows grow in most temperate zones of the world.

USES *Willow is also used to fuel ecologically effective and sustainable heating systems, as it grows very fast and takes more CO_2 from the air when it grows than it releases when it is burned. It is a good charcoal-making plant. You can also steam the young leaves and eat them.*

Willow bark is an antiseptic anti-inflammatory and a mild pain-killer that reduces fevers. It is used for arthritis, headaches, and stomach inflammation. Avoid if you are allergic to aspirin.

SAMBUCUS SPP.
Elder

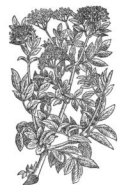

Sambucus nigra in Europe and *S. canadensis* in the United States is a small tree or large shrub. Common in Europe and North America, it produces creamy white clusters of small flowers, which develop into small, juicy, purple-black berries.

USES *The flowers and leaves increase sweating, are diuretic, and anti-inflammatory. They are used in teas, tinctures, and lotions for coughs and colds, and to treat arthritis and rheumatism.*

The berries are rich in vitamin C and are a powerful antiviral agent. They have a normalizing effect on the bowel and so can be used to help diarrhea, although they are also a mild laxative.

SCUTELLARIA LATERIFLORA
Skullcap

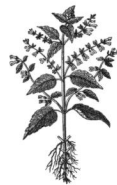

A perennial member of the mint family, this herb loves wet habitats. It has nettlelike leaves with serrated edges and blue-pink flowers. It is native to the United States and is cultivated in Europe.

USES *Skullcap is good for the nerves, and is widely used all over the world for almost any problem of the nervous system. It reduces anxiety, helps relaxation, and aids recovery from debility caused by long periods of overactivity and overwork. Related species are similarly used.*

SCUTELLARIA BAICALENSIS
Baical Skullcap—Huang Qin

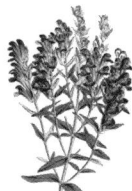

An herbaceous perennial from China with purple-blue flowers and lance-shape leaves, baical skullcap grows to 1–4 feet in height. In China, it is cultivated both as an ornamental plant and an important medicine. It is now also widely grown in the United States.

USES *The yellow root is one of Chinese medicine's fundamental herbs, used "to clear heat" from the body. An exceptional blood cleanser, it is useful for detoxing and for fighting infections—especially fevers of the lungs, throat, nose, and sinuses, when the mucus is thick and yellow.*

Baical skullcap stops bleeding and aids the healing of wounds. A liver tonic, it can be used in place of golden seal, which is endangered.

Do not use in pregnancy except under some form of professional supervision.

SALVIA OFFICINALIS AND SPP.
Common Sage

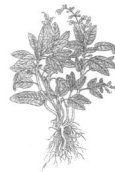

An aromatic flowering herb in the mint family, common sage has gray-green leaves and lilac flowers. It is a Mediterranean native, but is now widely naturalized.

USES *Sage is a culinary herb, delicious in savory dishes and salads.*

It is used all over the world as a medicine for infections, lung and digestive disorders, and skin problems. It is also an excellent general tonic for weakness and debility following illness.

Sage is a nourishing tonic for the brain and can relieve excessive sweating, including that occurring during menopause. Externally it helps to speed the healing of bruises and inflammations.

Do not take medicinal doses if pregnant (but as a spice in food it is fine), or if epileptic.

SILYBUM MARIANUM
Milk Thistle

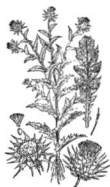

This robust, pink-purple-flowered thistle is native to Europe. It has prickly, variegated green and white leaves and can grow up to 5 feet tall. Milk thistle is widely cultivated, and its seeds have been used in healing for more than 2,000 years.

USES *Milk thistle seeds are a powerful healing agent for the liver, both protecting it from toxins and encouraging its regeneration. The herb is used to treat serious liver problems, including hepatitis and liver damage from drug and alcohol use. Milk thistle can be taken to protect the liver from the toxicity of medicines, including those used in medical treatment, but this can make medications less effective, because it speeds up their removal from the body. The ground seeds are commonly taken as capsules or tea.*

STACHYS OFFICINALIS
Wood Betony

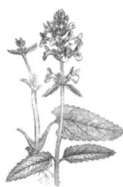

Also known as *Stachys betonica*, this perennial herb is native to grasslands in Europe, North Africa, and Asia. It has smallish, toothed leaves and clusters of purple flowers, on spikes that grow to 1–2 feet tall. It is cultivated in North America, where it is also known as hedgenettle, and sometimes is found naturalized.

USES *Wood betony is a powerful remedy for the stomach and the nervous system. It is a bitter tonic, especially beneficial for the brain. A tea or tincture is used to treat dizziness and dementia, as well as a sluggish liver, gallbladder problems, and poor digestion.*

Do not take during pregnancy.

SOLIDAGO SPP.
Goldenrod

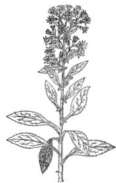

Native to the United States and introduced in Europe, goldenrod is an herbaceous perennial with a lovely spike of pollen-heavy yellow flowers.

USES *Goldenrod flowers, seeds, and leaves can be added to soups, stews, and stir-fries.*

It is a good tonic herb for the kidneys, even being used to treat serious problems, such as nephritis, and also supports the bladder and prostate.

Goldenrod is an anticatarrhal and anti-inflammatory tonic to the mucous membranes, used to treat the digestive system and chronic mucus in the nose, throat, and ears. It is taken as a tincture or tea.

STELLARIA MEDIA
Chickweed

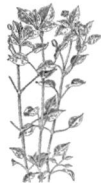

This creeping annual grows in the colder seasons in many locations in Europe and North America. Its Latin name comes from its tiny, star-shape white flowers, which peep out from its bright green leaves, shaped like mice's ears.

USES *Chickweed is tasty and nutritious, good to eat raw or lightly cooked; it is also great food for chickens. In herbal medicine, it is used for skin diseases and arthritis, and for bronchitis and lung disease. The plant is taken internally as a tea or tincture and externally as a cream, ointment, or infused oil.*

SYMPHYTUM OFFICINALE
Comfrey

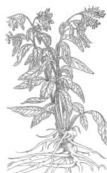

Comfrey thrives in damp and cool conditions. It has fleshy, dark green, hairy leaves and blue-purple, or sometimes white-pink, flowers. Its black roots conceal a white, gloopy (mucilaginous) interior.

USES *Also known as knitbone, comfrey considerably speeds the healing of connective tissue (ligaments, tendons, bones, and skin). It is used inside and out as tea and tincture, but the root is not taken internally because it contains pyrrolizidine alkaloids, toxic to the liver in large amounts.*

People with liver problems and those taking medications should avoid comfrey. Otherwise the leaves are fine for short-term use.

Do not use on open wounds because comfrey makes the skin heal so quickly it can heal over dirt or infection, tending to form raised scars.

TARAXACUM OFFICINALE
Dandelion

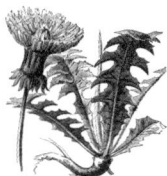

A common, yellow-flowered weed that grows every year from its deep root. Leaves are long and toothed, growing from a main flower stalk. The cluster of flowers later forms a seed head of hundreds of tiny seeds with fluffy hairs attached, enabling it to travel to new locations on the wind. It is native to Europe, Asia, and the Americas.

USES *The roots and leaves of dandelion are nutritious and used as foods and medicines everywhere the herb grows. Medicinally, the leaves are a powerful diuretic and kidney and liver tonic. The root is a strong liver tonic and stimulant, and a gentle laxative.*

Dandelion is used to detoxify and cleanse the body in treating skin and joint problems, cancers, headaches, and general weakness.

THUJA OCCIDENTALIS
White Cedar

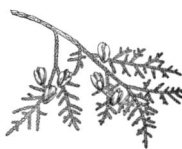

An evergreen in the cypress family bearing small cones, white cedar is native to eastern North America and grown in Europe as an ornamental plant. The branches, stem, and tiny, flat, scalelike leaves contain a strong essential oil.

USES *The plant is traditionally used to treat menstrual problems, headaches, and heart ailments.*

It is a diuretic used to relieve rheumatism and also helps catarrhal chest complaints. The herb is also used to reduce growths, including warts.

Liquid extracts, tinctures, and tea made from white cedar are taken internally in small doses (the tincture generally used at 1 tsp./5ml a week). The essential oil is used externally.

Do not take when pregnant or breastfeeding.

THYMUS SPP.
Thyme

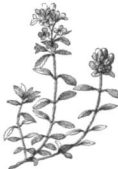

There are many species of this small-leaved, aromatic herb with woody stems and tiny pink flowers. *Thymus serpyllum*, or wild thyme, is native to southern Europe and a cultivated variety of this, *T. vulgaris*, is grown all around the world.

USES *Thyme contains an essential oil high in "thymol," a potent antiseptic. It is used against infections, particularly of the lungs and the digestive tract, including worms. Because it is relaxing for spasm, thyme is helpful for asthma and tight, aching muscles. It is a good general tonic.*

Do not use the essential oil when pregnant, and never take internally in any but the minutest amounts (and not even these if you have liver or kidney problems).

TRIFOLIUM PRATENSE
Red Clover

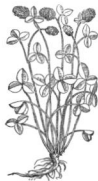

A beautiful, low-growing meadow flower with pink, globe-shape flower heads made of many tiny flowers. White markings decorate the 3-lobed leaves (occasionally you may find a 4-leaved clover, said to be lucky). It is native to Europe, Asia, and Africa and is naturalized in North America.

USES *This is a nourishing flower to eat any time, including during pregnancy. Red clover was traditionally used for coughs and respiratory problems, and also in treating cancer; it helps to stimulate the immune system into healthy functioning. The herb also has a mildly blood-thinning effect and is helpful for menopausal problems, such as hot flashes.*

Do not take red clover if you are on warfarin or other blood thinners.

UMBILICUS RUPESTRIS
Navelwort or Wall Pennywort

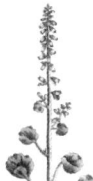

Native to Europe, navelwort grows on walls in shady places. It is a fleshy succulent with round leaves. The stem in the middle, which can be found all year round, is more prolific in the summer months when the flower spikes grow.

USES *It is delicious to eat and can be gathered in all seasons. Navelwort juice is cooling and eases pains, both taken internally and applied externally.*

Apply the juice or fresh poultice, or an ointment, to painful ears, painful hemorrhoids, wounds, gout, nerve pains, and sore throats. Take navelwort as a juice or tea for pains in the kidneys and digestive system.

TUSSILAGO FARFARA
Coltsfoot

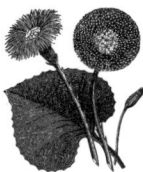

Coltsfoot is native to Europe, and can now be found in Canada and America's northeastern states. Its yellow dandelion-like flowers emerge in late winter to early spring. They then die down, and a month or so later the heart-shape gray-green leaves appear.

USES *Both the leaves and flowers of coltsfoot are an excellent expectorant and strengthening lung tonic.*

Like comfrey, it contains pyrrolizidine alkaloids, which in large amounts are toxic to the liver; therefore, coltsfoot is not recommended for long periods of use, nor for people with liver problems or those taking medications (because most of these are toxic to the liver).

Do not take while pregnant or breastfeeding.

URTICA DIOICA
Stinging Nettle

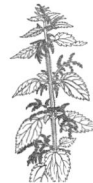

This perennial plant can grow more than 3 feet tall from its network of thin whitish roots, and has green, sharply serrated leaves. The undersides of the leaves are covered in fine, histamine-containing hairs which sting you if touched. It is native to Europe, United States, Asia, and North Africa.

USES *Nettles are one of the great panaceas of the plant world. Rich in minerals and vitamins and amino acids, in some countries they are one of the best, and easiest to find, wild plants to use as a food. The new green tops and the seeds are edible. Nettle leaves are used for arthritis, skin problems, and allergies, and are generally detoxifying and cleansing. Nettle root helps the prostate gland.*

VACCINIUM
Bilberry or Huckleberry

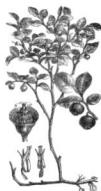

Bilberry is a low-growing, shrubby member of the heather family that grows on heaths, moors, and mountainous areas of Europe, Asia, and North America. It has small leaves and produces deep red-black fruits (resembling small blueberries).

USES *Bilberries are edible. The leaves and berries gathered before the berries ripen are used to protect eyesight and help with macular degeneration, cataracts, and diabetic eye problems. Bilberries can also help with high blood sugar, so are ideal for diabetics.*

Like other deep red-black fruits, the plant nourishes and helps to repair arteries and veins. Fresh berries are laxative, but dried ones are anti-infective and binding, so good for diarrhea. Leaves are also used to treat cystitis, kidney, and bladder complaints.

VERBASCUM THAPSUS
Mullein

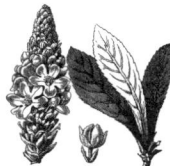

Native to Europe but naturalized in the United States, this beautiful herb has a tall spike of yellow flowers at its top and pale green-gray leaves. They feel as soft as velvet, being densely covered with fine hairs.

USES *Mullein is so rich in vitamins and minerals that it is a good herb to drink as tea regularly—although not very nice to eat because of its furriness.*

Mullein leaves and flowers soothe and calm inflamed lungs, helping deep and painful coughing, and ease the expectoration of mucus. They are also useful in treating hay fever and bed-wetting. Externally mullein is a good wound healer and helps to reduce piles. An oil made from the flowers is specific for earache.

It is used in smoking mixtures.

VALERIANA OFFICINALIS
Valerian

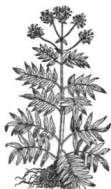

Every spring, this perennial begins to grow from a bundle of rhizome and thin roots to a tall, leafy plant, with flower heads of many small, pale, white and pinkish flowers. It prefers damp soil. It is native to Europe and northern Asia, but is much used in herbal medicine in the United States.

USES *The part of valerian used in medicine is the root and rhizome, and they have an extraordinary smell—you either love or hate it. Valerian is one of the most researched herbal sedatives and is used for anxiety, stress, insomnia, and physical tension. It is taken as a tea, pills, and tincture. Cats (including lions) adore it.*

Valerian can cause drowsiness and may react with sedative medication.

VERBENA SPP.
Vervain

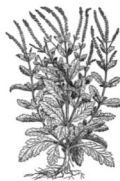

Vervain flowers form spikes of small, blue-purple blossoms. The European plant *V. officinalis* is spindly with purplish flowers, and its U.S. cousin, *V. hastate*, has sturdier stems and blue flowers. Both plants are used in similar ways.

USES *Vervain is a key herb for treating the nervous system. Herbalists value the plant as a relaxing nervine used for stress, tension, and nervous exhaustion. It is also a stimulating bitter tonic for the liver.*

Vervain was one of the most important plants of the Druids, being considered a powerful magical plant.

Do not use during pregnancy.

VIBURNUM OPULUS
Cramp Bark

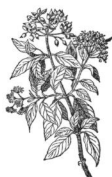

This deciduous shrub—also known as cranberry bush—is almost a tree, has vinelike leaves, white flowers, and red berries. It is native to the United States and Europe. An American cousin, *Viburnum prunifolium* (black haw), is also used in herbal medicine.

USES *As the name cramp bark suggests, this plant is a muscle relaxant and antispasmodic. Cramp bark is used to treat muscle cramps and tension, period pains and threatened abortion (it relaxes the womb), asthma (it relaxes spasm in the bronchial tubes of the lungs), colic, and spastic pains in the digestive tract. The herb also improves the circulation by opening blood vessels. Its American relative, black haw, is used similarly; it also treats morning sickness and problems in menopause.*

VITEX AGNUS-CASTUS
Chasteberry

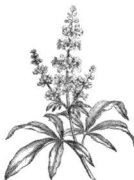

The tiny, yellow-red berries of this beautiful, aromatic Mediterranean flowering tree are known as "monkspepper" for its "an-aphrodisiac" effect—hence its other name of lilac chastetree.

USES *Chasteberry is used to treat premenstrual syndrome and menstrual irregularities, including those associated with menopause and polycystic ovarian syndrome. The plant can also help some women to conceive if infertility is caused by low progesterone levels, and it increases production of breast milk. Chasteberry can also be useful for acne and headaches associated with hormone imbalance, and can calm acne in teenage boys.*

VIOLA SPP.
Sweet Violet & Heartsease (Johnny-Jump-Up)

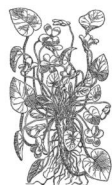

These two members of the violet family (*Viola odorata* and *V. tricolor*) are native to Europe and naturalized in the United States. Sweet violets have a delicious smell and are the traditional violet color. Heartsease is a "tricolor" pansy, with white, purple, and yellow flowers.

USES *Both herbs are used to treat bronchitis, asthma, and other lung problems. They are also useful for cystitis and an irritated bladder.*

Sweet violet helps to relieve congested lymph flow. It has also been used, internally and externally, in treating cancers and growths, both as a curative and a pain reliever.

Heartsease is particularly used for wet eczema and other skin diseases with sticky discharges.

ZINGIBER OFFICINALE
Ginger

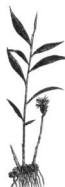

Ginger is widely known as a pungent culinary spice. The root of this relative of turmeric and cardamom originated in Asia, but is now used all over the world. It is a perennial plant resembling a reed, with lovely yellow flowers.

USES *Used in cooking savory and sweet dishes, as well as in pickles and confectioneries, ginger stimulates the whole system. The herb makes you sweat and so reduces fever, clears mucus from the head, sinuses, and lungs, and relaxes and stimulates the digestion, thus helping to treat indigestion, gas, and colic. Ginger helps to reduce nausea of all kinds, and is safe to take for morning sickness in pregnancy.*

It is also an excellent circulatory stimulant and can help to reduce high blood pressure.

CONTRIBUTORS

I offer grateful thanks to the following plant experts who have kindly shared their recipes.

Louise Berliner is an artist and writer from Massachusetts, who loves to play with herbs. See pp.*123, 154*

ChaNan Bonser practices creative kinesiology and runs "Elemental Medicine," offering physical therapy treatments in Wales, UK. See pp.*66, 174, 179*

Lynn-Amanda Brown is a multifaceted therapist and healer who works in alliance with the sacred energies of the natural world. She lives in Wales, UK. See p.*173*

Stephen Buhner is the award-winning author of 15 books on nature, indigenous cultures, the environment, and herbal medicine. He is one of the cofounders of The Foundation for Gaian Studies, an organization that explores and promotes our reconnection with Nature. He lives in New Mexico. See pp.*120, 170*

Anne Chiotis is an herbalist based in Wolverhampton, UK. See p.*80*

Sharon Cohen is a native plant expert living in the forests of Maryland. She runs Native Design, a company providing heart-base ecological restoration and garden design. See p.*141*

Michael Cole is a UK forager passionate about making leafu—a protein-rich food made from nettles and other edible wild greens. See p.*57*

Rachel Corby is a gardener, forager, and writer based in Stroud, UK. She runs Gateways to Eden, offering treatments and running workshops on the power of plants. See pp.*53, 163*

Eliot Cowan developed Plant Spirit Medicine and lives at the Blue Deer Center, New York State. He travels widely, teaching, healing, and promoting a balanced relationship with the human and other-than-human worlds. See pp.*85, 86*

Lesley Cunningham knows a lot about treating her horse friends with herbs. See pp.*138, 139*

Anna Dowding is a true domestic alchemist from North Wales, UK, who invents brilliant lotions and potions and coruns Getafix first aid and wild water sports experiences. See p.*131*

Geoff Edwards was an herbalist for many years and now runs UK-based t'ai chi center Wutan Bournemouth. See p.*99*

Teri Evans is a medical herbalist and runs Cunnynge Herbs in Shropshire, UK. Here, she sells artisan herbal tinctures and holds workshops on using herbs. See pp.*27, 33, 38, 64, 76, 88, 130, 178, 179, 180, 181, 182, 184, 185, 187, 189, 190, 191, 192, 201, 202, 203, 205, 207, 209, 210, 211, 214*

Annie Gardner is an herbalist based in Totnes, UK. See p.*152*

Monika Ghent is an herbalist and a Plant Spirit Medicine Healer. She runs Dreaming Willow natural therapies in Toronto, Canada, and designs and makes natural skin-care products. See pp.*77, 132, 183, 184, 188, 190, 192, 193, 209, 212*

Lucy Harmer is an international author and teacher based in Geneva, Switzerland. She is also a feng shui and space clearing expert, and a

high priestess on the Celtic Shamanic Path.
See pp.*36, 59, 186, 217, 218, 219*

Shelley Harrison is a healer and yoga teacher based near Ottawa, Canada.
See p.*152*

Christine Herren-Valette is a Swiss herbalist who trained as a medical nurse. She now runs a successful small business, Sancta Herba, making herbal products.
See pp.*63, 114, 175, 193*

Johanna Herzog is an herbalist and Plant Spirit Medicine practitioner. She runs a school of medicinal plants, or Heilkraeuterausbildung, near Hamburg, Germany.
See pp.*64, 74, 191, 208*

Wizz Holland is a Plant Spirit Medicine healer, forager, fire keeper, and animal communicator. Also a poet and artist, she is based in Devon, UK.
See pp.*55, 56, 145*

Louise Idoux is a medical herbalist from Shropshire, UK. She runs the Oswestry Herbarium, providing treatments and courses on making herbal products.
See pp.*61, 78, 96, 102, 136*

Catherine Johnson is a consulting medical herbalist in Wales, UK.
See pp.*89, 122*

Barbara Jones is an experienced veterinary surgeon who runs Vet Holistic in Shropshire, UK.
See pp.*135, 136, 137, 138*

Steve Kippax is an herbalist and TCM practitioner. He is Head of Complementary Medicine at The Third Space Medicine, London's leading integrated medical center.
See pp.*96, 102*

Dedj Leibbrandt is an herbalist and teacher in Hampshire, UK. Dedj was awarded a Fellowship of the National Institute of Medical Herbalists

for her work on acute medicine and herbal first aid.
See pp.*70, 82, 91, 101, 103, 106, 111, 121, 122, 135, 139*

Marc Luyckx is a domestic alchemist in Switzerland.
See p.*48*

Anne McIntyre is an experienced herbalist, plant grower, writer, and teacher, based in the Cotswolds, UK.
See pp.*107, 110, 114, 126, 127, 128, 129, 140, 153, 177*

Neil McNulty is an herbalist, iridologist, and facilitator who lives in Zagreb, Croatia. His practice is called Herba Vitalis, and his healing sanctuary is called "Wild at Heart."
See p.*62*

Alaina Mecklenburgh is a master herbalist practicing in the southern part of the Lake District in the UK.
See p.*213*

Joe Nasr is a medical herbalist, osteopath, and senior lecturer in herbal medicine, as well as a dedicated and experienced plant distiller. In 1997, Joe founded Avicenna, a company producing unique, high-quality herbal products in Wales, UK.
See pp.*65, 133*

Jenny Pao is a holistic health practitioner and aromatherapist. She runs Nectar Essences, a company based in San Francisco.
See pp.*180*

Annie Powell runs the Little Green Cream Company, a small ethical company making top-quality skin-care products in Wales, UK.
See pp.*66, 171, 177*

Lynn Rawlinson is a consulting medical herbalist and holistic therapist. She lives and works in Merseyside, UK.
See pp.*53, 118, 120, 181, 201, 202*

Anna Richardson runs wild food foraging courses for Circle of Life Rediscovery, UK, and is a Forest School leader and author.
See pp.*140, 141*

Melissa Ronaldson is a UK-based herbalist with a passion for snuff. She is cofounder of the Herbal Snuff Company.
See p.*124*

Jeanne Rose is an aromatherapist in San Francisco. She runs "The Aromatic Plant Project" and is the director and principal tutor of the Institute of Aromatic Studies.
See p.*57*

Anthony Seifert is a Californian herbalist who is on the faculty at the Ohlone Center for Herbal Studies in Berkeley, CA. He works with both humans and animals, and also runs an herbal supply company, Great Blue Heron Botanical Medicine Making Project.
See p.*114*

Sensory Solutions is a UK-based company run by traditional herbalists Karen Lawton and Fiona Heckels. They teach, grow, and collect plants to produce beautiful, high-quality remedies.
See pp.*75, 108, 164, 165*

Maida Silverman is an expert on wild plants that grow in New York City, where she has lived all her life.
See p.*179*

Tanya Smart runs the Yemoya company in Glastonbury, Somerset, UK, which makes the best organic soaps ever.
See pp.*196, 198*

Karen Stephenson has created and runs Edible Wild Foods, a wonderful website about foraging and eating wild food. She lives in Ontario, Canada.

See pp.*121, 143, 146, 149, 154, 155, 156, 157, 158, 160, 163, 164, 165, 203*

Iain Stewart is an herbalist working with the Rhizome Community Clinic in Bristol, UK.
See p.*80*

Sucandra devi dasi is a domestic alchemist from Hertfordshire, UK.
See p.*144*

Kamala Todd is an artist based in Malvern, UK, who makes rose petal bead jewelry.
See p.*215*

Michael Vertolli is a Western traditional herbalist who lives in Ontario, Canada. He is the founder and director of the Living Earth School of Herbalism.
See pp.*26, 92*

Emma Warrener is an herbalist in Lincolnshire, UK. She runs Herbs for Health and Wellbeing.
See pp.*195, 206*

Susun Weed is an herbalist and teacher based in Woodstock, NY. She is the voice of the Wise Woman Way.
See pp.*48, 149, 170*

Lucy Wells is a plant spirit medicine practitioner and fire keeper based in Shropshire, UK.
See pp.*57, 76*

Neil Williams is an herbalist who practices in the northwest of England, UK.
See pp.*98, 120*

Sue Wine is a McTimoney chiropractic based in Chester, Cheshire, UK.
See pp.*63, 87, 150*

Mathew Wood is a professional member of the American Herbalist's Guild and the author of six books on herbal medicine. He lives in Oregon.
See pp.*18-19, 116, 117*

SOURCES & FURTHER READING

Books

Bartram, Thomas, 1995. *The Encyclopedia of Herbal Medicine* (Dorset: Grace Publishers)

Bond, Annie B., 2005. *Home Enlightenment* (Kindle edition)

Buhner, Stephen Harrod, 2004. *The Secret Teachings of Plants* (Vermont: Bear & Company)

Buhner, Stephen Harrod, 2002. *The Lost Language of Plants* (Vermont: Chelsea Green Publishing)

Buhner, Stephen Harrod, 1998. *Sacred and Herbal Healing Beers* (Boulder: Siris Books)

Chevallier, Andrew, 1996–2000. *Encyclopedia of Herbal Medicine* (London: Dorling Kindersley)

Corby, Rachel and Studd, Stephen, 2009. *The Medicine Garden* (Preston: The Good Life Press)

Cowan, Eliot, 2014. *Plant Spirit Medicine* (Boulder: Sounds True)

Dau Dayal das, 2014. *The Beautiful Song of God – Srimad Bhagavad Gita* (Llangollen: The Dreaming Butterfly)

Hawes, Zoe, 2010. *Wild Drugs: A Forager's Guide to Healing Plants* (London: Gaia)

Hedley, Christopher and Shaw, Non, 1996. *Non Herbal Remedies: A Practical Beginner's Guide to Making Effective Remedies in the Kitchen* (Bristol: Parragon)

Hoffman, David, 1990. *Holistic Herbal: A Safe and Practical Guide to Making and Using Remedies* (Shaftesbury: HarperCollins)

Hughes, Nathaniel and Owen, Fiona, 2014. *Intuitive Herbalism* (Stroud: Quintessence)

Jeffery, Josie, 2011. *Seedbombs – Going Wild With Flowers* (Lewes: Leaping Hare Press)

McIntyre, Anne, 2011. *Drugs in Pots* (London: Gaia)

Michael, Pamela, 1986. *A Country Harvest* (London: Peerage Books)

Silverman, Maida, 1997. *A City Herbal* (Woodstock: Ash Tree Publishing)

Waller, Pip, 2009. *Holistic Anatomy—An Integrative Guide to the Human Body* (Berkeley: North Atlantic Books)

Weisse, Vivien, 2002. *The Gourmet Weed Cookery Book* (Norderstedt: VIWO)

Wood, Matthew, 1997. *The Book of Herbal Wisdom* (Berkeley: North Atlantic Books)

Yasodananda das, 2013. *Kitchen of Love* (Haarlem: Bhaktimedia.org)

Useful Websites

www.pipwaller.co.uk (my professional website)

www.thedomesticalchemist.com.org (for herbal news and my latest recipes)

www.americanherbalistsguild.com (for finding an herbalist in the United States)

www.anamed.net (for growing *Artemisia annua* in the Tropics)

www.ediblewildfood.com (for great foraging information and recipes)

www.gaianstudies.org (for U.S.-based training from The Foundation for Gaian Studies)

www.globalhealingcenter.com (for information about growing plants in the United States)

www.herbnet.com (for everything herbal in the United States)

www.herbworld.com (for an online encyclopedia with herbal information)

www.mercola.com (for a health information and research site in the United States)

www.nimh.org.uk (the National Institute of Medical Herbalists: for finding a UK herbalist)

www.wddty.com (What Doctors Don't Tell You: A site with interesting reviews of research)

INDEX

ACKNOWLEDGMENTS

I would like to thank the many people who have made this book possible.

A huge thank you to all at Leaping Hare, particularly the lovely Monica Perdoni who spotted me during my two-minute *Countryfile* appearance and had the idea for *The Herbal Handbook for Home and Health*, and Jayne Ansell who is a tirelessly patient editor. Also thanks to the art director, Wayne Blades, and designer, Andrew Milne, for making a beautiful book.

Thanks to my parents, Sheila and David Waller, who got me into herbal medicine in the first place by their example, and for all their help and support over the years.

Thanks to my beloved Dauji for his loving support and clever suggestions, my son Alex and my friends who tried a lot of weird and wonderful recipes— some that made it, some that didn't—and listened to a lot of gnashing of teeth as I wrestled with the computer over this project.

Thanks to all the fabulous herbalists, plant spirit medicine practitioners, and plant lovers who generously gave their recipes—you have made this book the interesting and varied mixture of recipes that it is. Thanks also to those whose recipes were too long for this volume—I'm hoping to feature yours in volume two!

Thanks to Louise for letting me loose with my cups and spoons in the Herbarium shop and helping me get to grips with U.S./European measuring eccentricities.

Thanks to my friends in the plant world, the herbs themselves, for calling to me again and again and waving to me wherever I go.

And last but not least, thank you Radharani, for being the One who is behind everything.

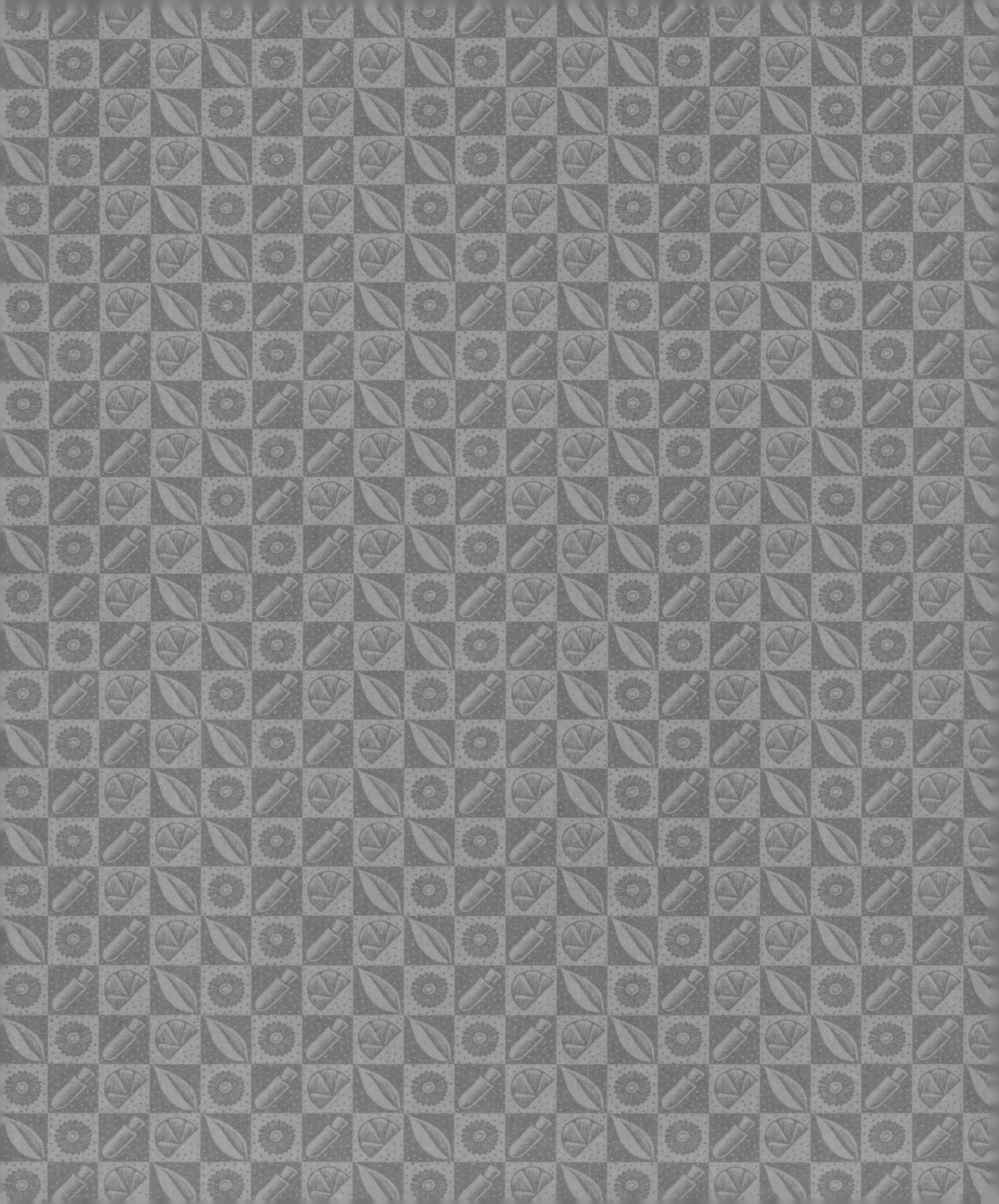